Vertigo

Advance Praise for *Vertigo*

"I read this book from cover to cover and found it engaging, enlightening, and inspiring. It has many revealing vignettes about the personal lives of the giants in neuro-otology whose eponymous names we all recognize. Bob Baloh's story illustrates how science, and especially medicine, moves forwards, sideways, backwards, and then often belatedly, forwards again. And the book points out, as always, the human failings of even our most brilliant scientific heroes; jealousy, selective memory, and an unwillingness to give up one's own theories in the face of incontrovertible opposing evidence. Lessons for us all."

—**David S. Zee, MD**, Professor, Neuro-Visual & Vestibular Division, Departments of Neurology, Ophthalmology, Otolaryngology-Head and Neck Surgery, and Neuroscience, The Johns Hopkins Hospital, Baltimore, MD

"A riveting account by one of the giants in the field, of how clinician-scientists, have managed over the last century to unravel the secrets of the sixth sense, the sense of motion and to apply their findings to the treatment of balance disorders to give relief to those suffering from terrifying vertigo attacks. Full of fascinating information for both patients and professionals—a must read."

—**Michael Halmagyi, BSC, MBBS, MD**, Royal Prince Alfred Hospital, Sydney, Australia

"A fascinating story of scientific discovery. Mysterious and disabling spinning sensations, psychoanalysis, pigeons, the Nobel prize, imprisonment in Russia, exile to Sweden, bouncing eyes, ear stones, and a simple but elusive cure. Dr. Baloh, a giant in the field himself, tells the story like no one else could."

—**Kevin Kerber, MD**, Department of Neurology, University of Michigan, Ann Arbor, MI

"The sense of balance was one of the first sensory systems to emerge in evolution, but it was also the last to be discovered. In his remarkable book *Vertigo: Five Physician Scientists and the Quest for a Cure*, Robert W. Baloh transports the reader back to the early days of vestibular discoveries, exemplified by five eminent figures in the history of neurotology. Dr. Baloh brings to life the colorful personalities that deepened our understanding of the balance system and paved the way for current vestibular diagnostics and treatment. This meticulously researched book, written by an eminent specialist in the field, will make a significant contribution to the history of vestibular science."

—**Gerald Wiest, MD**, Professor of Neurology, Medical University Vienna, Vienna, Austria

Vertigo

Five Physician Scientists and the Quest for a Cure

ROBERT W. BALOH, MD
Professor of Neurology and Head and Neck Surgery
David Geffen School of Medicine at UCLA
Director of the Neurotology Clinic and Laboratory
Ronald Regan Medical Center
Los Angeles, CA

OXFORD
UNIVERSITY PRESS

OXFORD
UNIVERSITY PRESS

Oxford University Press is a department of the University of Oxford. It furthers
the University's objective of excellence in research, scholarship, and education
by publishing worldwide. Oxford is a registered trade mark of Oxford University
Press in the UK and certain other countries.

Published in the United States of America by Oxford University Press
198 Madison Avenue, New York, NY 10016, United States of America.

© Oxford University Press 2017

Library of Congress Cataloging-in-Publication Data
Names: Baloh, Robert W. (Robert William), 1942– author.
Title: Vertigo : five physician scientists and the quest for a cure / by Robert W. Baloh.
Description: Oxford ; New York : Oxford University Press, [2017] |
Includes bibliographical references and index.
Identifiers: LCCN 2016021216 | ISBN 9780190600129 (alk. paper)
Subjects: | MESH: Vertigo—history | Benign Paroxysmal Positional
Vertigo—therapy | Physicians | Biography
Classification: LCC RB150.V4 | NLM WB 143 | DDC 616.8/4106—dc23
LC record available at https://lccn.loc.gov/2016021216

1 3 5 7 9 8 6 4 2

Printed by Sheridan Books, Inc., United States of America

CONTENTS

PREFACE

My interest in the history of neurotology began early in my career in the mid-1970s after a series of conversations with Raphael Lorente de Nó. My longtime friend and collaborator, Vicente Honrubia, was instrumental in bringing Lorente to UCLA, where he spent the last 5 years of his academic career before retiring to Arizona. Lorente told fascinating stories of his time in Uppsala, Sweden, with Robert Bárány. During the next 20 years, I maintained my interest by reading and collecting historical material, but my focus was on my research career. In the late 1990s, my interest in the history of neurotology was rekindled by a young neurologist, Gerald Wiest, who came to work in my lab as a visiting researcher from Vienna, Austria. Gerald not only had an interest in the history of neurotology but also had access to key documents at the University of Vienna library, many of which had not been previously translated into English.

In the early 2000s, I wrote a series of articles focusing on five physician scientists who stood out among the many working in the field: Prosper Ménière, Josef Breuer, Robert Bárány, Charles Hallpike, and Harold Schuknecht. Each made major scientific discoveries and each had a compelling personal story. Journal articles, by nature, must be highly focused, and in my research I collected a large amount of material including personal interviews that I saved for publication at a later date.

At approximately the same time, I became interested in the story of the discovery of a simple cure for benign paroxysmal positional vertigo (BPPV). It became clear to me that in many ways the history of the discovery of a cure for BPPV was a microcosm of the history of neurotology. It certainly was the crowning achievement of research in the field. The five physician scientists mentioned previously were key players in the story, with each representing a different era in the history of neurotology. Furthermore, because I was involved in the research on BPPV, I knew the recent key players personally and was able to interview them.

This book provides a historical approach to understanding the anatomy and physiology of the vestibular system—the parts of the inner ear involved in balance and equilibrium and their connections within the brain. I hope it will be of interest to anyone who has experienced vertigo, particularly if they have an interest in science or the history of science. It will be of particular interest to neuroscientists who work on the vestibular system; to physicians, audiologists, and therapists who specialize in treating patients with vertigo; and to students who want to learn about the vestibular system. I strongly believe that the best way to develop a foundation of knowledge in any field is to understand the historical development in that field. I am interested in the people who made the important discoveries. What are they like? What motivates them? What did they think about their accomplishments? As with all areas of science, there is a jargon that goes with the field, and I have attempted to minimize the impact of the jargon as much as possible by defining terms as they are introduced and providing a glossary and a "map" of the ear in the beginning of the first chapter. Numerous illustrations are used to clarify difficult concepts.

Although I use BPPV as a unifying theme for the book, there are many "side trips" into basic anatomy and physiology of the vestibular system and into historical and biographical sketches. I hope the reader will bear with me and find these "side trips" interesting in their own right but also helpful in providing a background for understanding the journey to a cure for BPPV.

ACKNOWLEDGMENTS

I thank Vicente Honrubia, Rinaldo Canalis, John Mazziotta, and my other colleagues in Head and Neck Surgery and Neurology who, throughout the years, provided support and encouragement. I also thank my fellows and trainees who provided the inspiration to learn and discover. Gerald Wiest, my colleague from Vienna, Austria, provided invaluable assistance in obtaining and translating key documents. Gerald reviewed the manuscript and provided helpful suggestions. Michael Halmagyi, my friend and colleague from Sydney, Australia, also read the manuscript and had useful comments. Finally, I thank Craig Panner at Oxford University Press for believing in the project and helping with the editing.

Introduction

The Inner Ear

The ear is made up of three separate structures: the outer ear consisting of the ear lobe and external auditory canal; the middle ear, a cavity on the other side of the ear drum containing tiny bones (ossicles) that conduct sound from the outer to the inner ear; and the inner ear, also called the labyrinth, where the sensory receptors for balance and hearing reside (Figure 1.1). The inner ear is a remarkable organ. It is only the size of the tip of one's little finger, yet it contains three major sensory receptors: the crista of the semicircular canals for sensing angular acceleration, the macule of the utricle and saccule for sensing linear acceleration, and the organ of Corti of the cochlea for sensing sound (straight arrows in the lower half of Figure 1.1). You will probably want to refer back to Figure 1.1 as these terms are discussed frequently throughout the text. They are all defined in the glossary.

The hearing function of the inner ear was known for centuries, but its role in balance and equilibrium was only discovered approximately a century and a half ago when a French physician working at a deaf-mute institute in Paris, Prosper Ménière, noted that patients with damage to the inner ear often had a combination of vertigo and hearing loss. Prior to that time, a patient with vertigo (regardless of the cause) was said to have "cerebral congestion," a condition resulting from excessive blood filling the brain whereby "bleeding" and leeches were the treatment of choice to relieve the congestion.

Dizziness, Vertigo, and the Inner Ear

In everyday English, "vertigo" is often misused in a nonspecific manner to refer to a dizzy confused state of mind such as the disoriented sensation that many normal people experience with heights made famous in the Alfred Hitchcock movie *Vertigo*. Just about everyone has experienced a brief lightheaded dizzy sensation after jumping up rapidly from a lying or sitting position. This usually

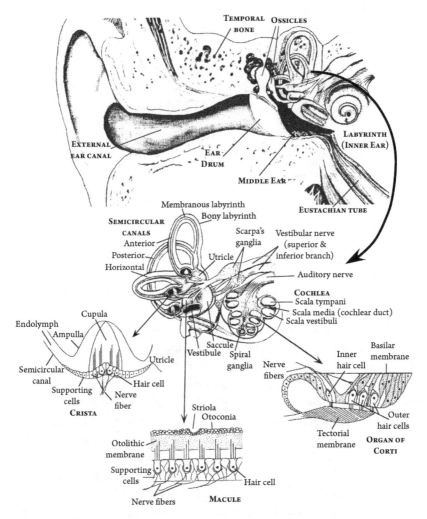

Figure 1.1 ANATOMY OF THE EAR WITH EMPHASIS ON THE INNER EAR.
IMPORTANT STRUCTURES ARE DEFINED IN THE GLOSSARY AND THROUGHOUT
THE TEXT.

results from brief drops in blood pressure upon standing. These are examples of
dizziness but not vertigo.

Dizziness is a broad, catch-all term used for any sensation of disorientation.
It encompasses vertigo but also a range of other abnormal sensations, including giddiness, lightheadedness, and a near-faint sensation. Vertigo is derived
from a Latin word meaning to turn or whirl, and its medical definition is that of
an illusion of movement—usually spinning or turning but occasionally linear
movement or tilt. Because one of the main functions of the inner ear is to sense
movement of the head, abnormalities of the inner ear or its connections in the
brain cause an illusion of movement—vertigo.

What Is Benign Paroxysmal Positional Vertigo?

Benign paroxysmal positional vertigo (BPPV) is by far the most common cause of vertigo. Approximately one in five people will experience it during their lifetime. Sudden violent spells of spinning are triggered by a change in position such as turning over in bed, getting in and out of bed, and extending the head back to look up. Often there is associated nausea and vomiting. These vertigo attacks are frightening particularly when they first occur because people often think they are having a stroke or another life-threatening condition. Between the attacks, there may be a residual motion sick sensation that persists throughout the day. During the attacks, both eyes oscillate, a phenomena called nystagmus. As discussed later, the characteristic appearance of the nystagmus during an attack of BPPV was key to understanding the cause.

There are few things in medicine that have as dramatic an impact on both the patient and the physician as the curative procedure for BPPV. Patients are not used to simple answers for terrifying symptoms such as vertigo. After I am sure of the diagnosis, I explain to patients that they are suffering from a common problem in which tiny particles have inappropriately entered one of the semicircular canals in the inner ear. There is a simple procedure to cure it. Upon hearing this, most patients envision some type of surgical procedure to remove the tiny particles. When I explain that it can be accomplished by simply extending their head over the back of the table and turning it across to the other side, most are skeptical. Once I convince them to perform the positioning maneuver and they do not have positional vertigo when they extend their head back a second time, they begin to accept my story. The real accolades do not come until approximately 1 week later, however, when they are finally convinced that they are cured.

So where do these tiny particles come from and where do they go? The particles are calcium carbonate crystals (otoconia) attached to a membrane in one of the chambers of the inner ear, the utricle (see Figure 1.1). The weight of these tiny particles on a specialized sensory organ in the membrane (the macule) provides the brain with a signal regarding the direction of gravity, the direction of up and down. The particles can be dislodged with a blow to the head or after any kind of damage to the inner ear, but they can also dislodge and float free for no apparent reason, particularly in older people. Once the particles are freely floating in the inner ear fluid they can enter one of the semicircular canals, particularly if the head is tilted backward. Once they are in the semicircular canal, they move with changes in position, triggering a signal to the brain that a person is spinning in the plane of the canal. The previously mentioned curative maneuver simply allows these particles to roll out of the semicircular canal into the larger chamber (the utricle), where they are normally attached to the sensory organ and where they can no longer cause symptoms.

What happens to the particles once they have left the semicircular canal? This is not entirely clear, although they probably either dissolve in the fluid or are taken up into the membrane (a process called phagocytosis). In some people, they remain freely floating and can re-enter the semicircular canal, particularly if the head is tilted far back to extreme positions. That is why patients are told to avoid extending their head far back after undergoing the treatment maneuver.

Who Discovered the Cure?

It is difficult to say who exactly deserves credit for discovery of this dramatic cure. As with most discoveries in medicine, there is a long list of contributors, each providing a small piece to the puzzle. As I began to delve into the history of the discovery, I became intrigued with five amazing individuals who made the major contributions. The road to the discovery of a cure for BPPV involved investigators from around the world and was strewn with missed opportunities, serendipitous findings, and academic intrigue, no different than that of most other medical discoveries. Knowing what we know today, most of the observations seem simple. Anybody could have made them. All of the key information for understanding the mechanism and even a cure for BPPV was present at the beginning of the 20th century, yet nearly another century passed before all the pieces of the puzzle were properly put together and the simple cure was developed and accepted. In this book, I tell the story of how the cause of BPPV was discovered and how the simple bedside cure was developed.

PROSPER MÉNIÈRE (1799–1862)

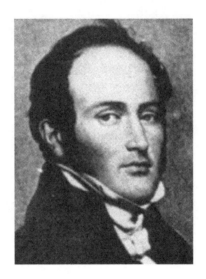

In the mid-19th century, Paris was the center of the newly developing science of medicine. Louis Pasteur reported his classical experiments on fermentation before the Academy of Sciences in 1859. He would soon prove his germ theory of disease—the idea that diseases could be caused by outside infective organisms rather than by humors, miasmas, and other vague factors. The famous physiologist Claude Bernard demonstrated how the body made, stored, and metabolized a form of sugar that he called glycogen. He found that even if animals were fed no sugar, they synthesized sugar in the liver in the form of glycogen. Jean Martin Charcot, the father of modern neurology, was appointed chief of the medical services at the Salpetriere, where he would systematically describe most of the common neurologic diseases. In 1861, Prosper Ménière presented his famous paper on vertigo and hearing loss before the Imperial Academy of Medicine.

Ménière Recognizes That Vertigo Can Originate from the Inner Ear

As director of a large deaf-mute institute in Paris, it is not difficult to understand how Prosper Ménière concluded that vertigo results from diseases of the inner ear. He undoubtedly saw many patients with the combination of vertigo and deafness. What is difficult, however, is to appreciate how controversial this concept was when he first presented it. At that time, the role of the inner ear as an organ of hearing was known, but its role in maintaining balance and orientation was completely unknown.

The symptom of vertigo originally fell under the rubric of apeplectiform cerebral congestion, a disorder thought to result from overfilling of blood vessels in the brain. Treatment consisted of bleeding, leeching, cupping, and purging—a regimen that required a hardy constitution to withstand. Based on his experience, Ménière noted that patients with vertigo and associated hearing loss often have a benign course and aggressive treatments such as bleeding can be more dangerous than the underlying disease. Knowing what we know today, this seems straightforward common sense, but in 1861 it was considered heretical (Baloh, 2001).

What Was Known About the Inner Ear in the Mid-19th Century?

The concept that diseases could originate from a single organ such as the inner ear was just beginning to be accepted by the medical community in the 19th century. The influence of Hippocrates and Galen still dominated the practice of medicine. These ancients believed that diseases acted throughout the body and were due to disturbances of four humors—black bile, yellow bile, phlegm, and blood. In essence, the theory held that disease resulted from either a deficit or an excess of one of these humors and good health required the humors to be in balance. This theory gave rise to bloodletting, leeches, and many of the other treatments described later in this chapter. It was not until the mid-16th century that detailed dissections of the human body were made and the concept of organ-specific disease began to evolve. Galen had written extensively on anatomy, but his writings were full of errors because he had never actually dissected a human. In 1543, Vasalius, the first in a long line of great anatomists to study and work at the University of Padua in Italy (Pappas, 1996), published his monumental *De Humani Corporis Fabrica* that for the first time provided an accurate description of the organs of the human body. To give some idea of how ingrained Galen's teachings were within the medical community, a contemporary of Vasalius, Jacques du Bois of Amiens, remarked that any structure found in contemporary man that differed from Galen's description could only be due to a "decadence and degeneration in mankind" (Talbott, 1970).

Gabriel Falloppio (Falloppius) succeeded Vasalius in Padua in 1551 and provided the first detailed description of the anatomy of the ear. He described the shape and features of the eardrum and middle ear and was the first to direct attention to the semicircular canals in the inner ear (see Figure 1.1). He is most famous for describing the canal housing the facial nerve (Fallopian canal) that he noted resembled an aqueduct.

Antonio Mario Valsalva provided the first description of the anatomy of the inner ear in 1704. Valsalva was part of the great University of Bologna tradition that began with his mentor Malpighi, his own student Morgagni, and finally Cotugno, who discovered the fluid of the inner ear (perilymph) in 1760. Another Italian physician, Antonio Scarpa, provided the first detailed description of the membranous structure of the inner ear.

Scarpa is probably best known for his description of the vestibular nerve ganglia because it was named after him, Scarpa's ganglia (see Figure 1.1), but he published extensively on the microanatomy of the inner ear in a wide range of animals. He was born in Treviso in the Republic of Venice in 1752 and was tutored in mathematics, philosophy, and Latin by his uncle, an enlightened priest. Scarpa initially planned to be a priest himself but later decided on a career in medicine. He entered the University of Padua at age 15, graduated with honors at age 19, and published his first work at age 20. The article titled "Anatomical Observations on the Structure of the Round Window of the Ear, or Second Tympanum" led to a long dispute with the famous Italian physician, biologist, and physicist, Luigi Galvani, who claimed that some of Scarpa's findings were identical to research that he had published previously. Scarpa eventually won the ascendancy battle and in the process demonstrated the ruthlessness and political savvy that propelled his academic career (Canalis et al., 2001).

In 1781, after traveling and working in Vienna, Paris, and London, Scarpa was appointed chair of anatomy at the well-respected University of Pavia through the intervention of the chief physician to the Emperor Joseph II. Scarpa's accomplishments in research and surgery brought him to the attention of Maria Teresa, archduchess of Austria, who provided funds for a state-of-the-art anatomy theater named in his honor. Napoleon Bonaparte appointed Scarpa surgeon to his court. Later in his career, Scarpa became a wealthy man and acquired a large collection of Renaissance paintings. His colleagues considered him aloof probably because of his single-minded pursuit of recognition and power. He never married but had many romantic affairs and at least one illegitimate son whose tragic death triggered a period of depression. After he retired in 1813, he lived in the hills of Pavia, where he died alone and friendless. In his will, he directed one of his former assistants to sever his head so that it could be preserved for posterity. It now resides at the historical museum of the University of Pavia.

Scarpa published a wide range of scientific publications during his long tenure at the University of Pavia, many of which are considered medical classics. His most significant publication related to the ear was *Anatomical Investigations on Hearing and Smell*, published by the Italian publisher Pietro Galeatti, Pavia, in 1780. The Latin version was reprinted four times during the next 14 years. (An excellently preserved copy of the first edition is part of the rare books collection at UCLA.)

The first section *Anatomical Investigations* focuses on the ears of insects, worms, fish, reptiles, and birds; the second section deals with the human ear; and the third section describes the olfactory organ of fish, reptiles, birds, and humans. For his study of the human inner ear, he relied on a high-quality magnifying lens (×9) because microscopes were still crude and not very versatile at that time. Scarpa was well aware that inside the dense bony capsule there was a membranous organ similar to the ones he had seen in his animal work (Scarpa, 1789):

> The membranous canals are disposed within the axis of the osseous tubes in such a way that they are invariably held secure in their center by a most tenuous web. . . . In fact, the membranous tubes are notably narrower than the diameter of the bony canals, appearing throughout and anywhere one looks quite free and loose within the surrounding bone. (pp. 44–45)

Scarpa preferred to study fresh human specimens because he knew that the delicate membranous structures he was attempting to study would rapidly deteriorate after death. He used a range of saws, trepans, scalpels, gauges, and knives for the delicate dissection. The plates for the illustrations in Scarpa's book were etched by the well-known engraver, Faustino Anderioni, based on Scarpa's own drawings (Figure 2.1) and were remarkably detailed and accurate for their time.

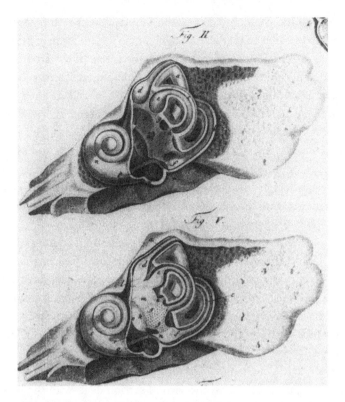

Figure 2.1 Two figures illustrating the structure of the inner ear (labyrinth) from Antonio Scarpa's *Anatomicae disquisitiones de auditu et olfactu* (1789). The top figure (II) shows the bony capsule, and the bottom figure (V) shows the membranous semicircular canals, utricle, saccule, and cochlea inside the bony capsule. Source: Courtesy Rinaldo Canalis, MD, UCLA.

Legend has it that Scarpa locked Anderioni in his room until the illustrations were complete.

Interestingly, despite Scarpa's detailed anatomical studies that clearly showed a functional separation between the cochlea and the vestibular part of the inner ear, he stuck with contemporary dogma and believed that the inner ear was exclusively an organ of hearing. It would take another half century before a balance function of the inner ear was recognized.

First Hint That the Semicircular Canals May Be Related to Balance

By the beginning of the 19th century, detailed anatomy was available on all parts of the ear, including the microanatomy of the inner ear. There was relatively little information about how the inner ear functioned. The cochlea was known to be an organ of hearing because damage to the cochlea resulted in hearing loss. In 1791, Carlos Mondini of the University of Bologna described malformation of the cochlea in a young deaf boy. The function of the semicircular canals, on the other hand, was largely unknown, although most believed that the canals had something to do with hearing, possibly localizing the direction of sound in three-dimensional space. A Frenchman, Marie Jean Pierre Flourens, provided the first insight into what the semicircular canals might be doing (Flourens, 1842). Like Scarpa, Flourens was a child prodigy, having enrolled at the famous Montpellier medical school in southern France at age 15 years and received his medical degree at age 19 years (Pearce, 2009). After studying brain function under Georges Cuvier in Paris, Flourens was asked to investigate Joseph Gall's popular theory of phrenology by the Paris Academy of Sciences acting on a request from Napoleon Bonaparte.

Franz Joseph Gall developed his theory of phrenology in Vienna in the late 18th century and moved to Paris in 1807 because of restrictions on teaching and publishing in Vienna (Ackerknecht and Vallois, 1956). Gall's theory was composed of four basic premises: (1) Moral and intellectual qualities are innate; (2) these qualities depend on brain function; (3) the brain is the organ of all faculties, of all tendencies, and of all feelings; and (4) the brain is composed of many organs because there are many faculties, tendencies, and feelings. Based on what we know today, these premises are reasonable, and if Gall had stopped there his place in history would be solid. However, he did not stop there. He went on to describe 27 brain centers (organs), each with specific functions, including centers for vanity, satire, sagacity, talent, kindness, and religion. Because he believed that the skull was "molded" to the brain, he thought it was possible to examine the shape of the brain by examining the shape of the skull (cranioscopy). Gall's skull palpating became extremely popular in progressive Parisian society, but like the Emperor of Austria, Napoleon saw antireligious materialistic ideas in Gall's teachings. And suffice it to say that Napoleon was not pleased with the rumor that his head was too small to lend itself to phrenological examination.

Flourens had a simple scheme to test Gall's brain localization theory. He systematically removed anatomically defined regions of the brains of animals and then observed the animals' behavior. With this technique, he showed that after damage to the cerebellum the animals could no longer coordinate movements, and after damage to the medulla of the brainstem, vital functions such as respiration were lost. However, he did not find evidence of cortical localization and concluded that the brain functioned as a whole: "A large section of the cerebral lobes can be removed without loss of function. As more is removed, all functions weaken and gradually disappear. Thus the cerebral lobes operate in unison for the full exercise of their function" (Changeux, 1985). Thus, Gall and Flourens began the battle of the "localizers" (Gall) versus the "generalizers" (Flourens) that raged throughout the latter half of the 19th century.

Flourens did his work mainly on pigeons and rabbits, which likely explains why he failed to recognize localization of cerebral cortical function. He never studied primates, in which cerebral localization is much easier to identify. On the other hand, because the inner ear is well developed and is easily accessible in pigeons, Flourens was better able to study the effect of selective ablation of different parts of the inner ear. He systematically cut each semicircular canal in the pigeon and noted that the animal's head and body tended to move in the plane of the damaged canal. Damage to the posterior semicircular canal caused the pigeon to fall backward, whereas destruction of the anterior semicircular canal caused the animal to fall forward. When the horizontal canal was damaged, the bird's head and body turned around a vertical axis. Flourens did not appreciate that the organs he was destroying were related to the animal's sense of equilibrium but, rather, he thought they were somehow involved in the control of movements in the pigeon. Flourens also studied the cochlea and was the first to conclusively prove that this was the only part of the inner ear involved in the perception of sound. Ménière was well aware of the work of Flourens, and in his classical 1861 paper, Ménière quoted it in support of his theory that vertigo could originate from the inner ear (Ménière, 1861b). The gyrations of the animals described by Flourens made Ménière think that vertigo in humans might be a similar phenomenon.

Ménière Presents His Findings in 1861

Ménière was 61 years old when he stepped up to the platform to present his famous paper on vertigo and the inner ear before the Imperial Academy of Medicine on January 8, 1861 (Ménière, 1861a). Surprisingly, the title of his presentation, "On a Particular Kind of Severe Hearing Loss Resulting from a Lesion of the Inner Ear," did not reflect his basic premise that vertigo could result from a lesion of the inner ear. Perhaps he was trying to avoid controversy. The title of the full paper published later that year, "A Report on Lesions of the Inner Ear Giving Rise to Symptoms of Cerebral Congestion of Apoplectic Type," was more to the point (Ménière, 1861b). Although Ménière was a well-respected physician in the Parisian medical community, he was not a member of the Academy. On two occasions, his name was brought before the body for a vote, but he did not receive an adequate number of votes for election. Not being a member of the Academy, he could not participate in the discussion after his presentation. This was not important, however, because it was a cold, rainy day and only a few members were in attendance (Atkinson, 1961). In fact, they showed little interest in his speculation about vertigo, deafness, and the inner ear. After all, deafness was known to be an incurable condition, and nothing much was known about the balance function of the inner ear.

The First Recorded Case of Ménière's Disease?

As noted previously, Ménière's presentation was first published in abstract form (Ménière, 1861a), and later in the year the full manuscript was published (Ménière, 1861b). Ménière began the manuscript by describing a clinical case with vertigo and hearing loss (as translated in Atkinson, 1961):

> A healthy young man would experience suddenly, without apparent cause, vertigo, nausea, vomiting; a condition of indescribable distress drained his strength; his face pale and bathed with sweat proclaimed approaching collapse . . . lying on his back he could not open his eyes without seeing the objects around him whirling in space; the slightest movement of the head increased the vertigo and nausea; vomiting started again as soon as the patient tried to change his position. (pp. 14–15)

These attacks came on abruptly during periods of perfect health without any apparent precipitating factor. Ménière went on to describe how even in between these spontaneous attacks of vertigo, the young man would have brief spells of positional vertigo when lying down in bed or when getting out of bed. If he got into bed rapidly (as translated in Atkinson, 1961),

> at-once the bed and all of the surrounding objects started upon a huge gyratory movement as though he were on the deck of a ship rolling through a wide arc, and nausea manifested itself at once just as at the beginning of sea sickness. (pp. 15–16)

The patient was given a diagnosis of cerebral congestion, and he was treated with the standard regimen of bleeding and purgatives. Even though these treatments were "accepted with eagerness," they had no effect on his symptoms. The patient then began noticing loud noises in his ears along with decreased hearing, first in one ear and then in both. Based on these new symptoms, Ménière concluded that the association of a "cerebral symptom," vertigo, and the auditory symptoms of tinnitus and hearing loss were due to a single disease (as translated in Atkinson, 1961):

> Although all the parts of the ear which could be studied directly or indirectly were free from abnormality, I could not forget that beyond the

> middle ear there exists an apparatus [the inner ear] which, mysterious as it
> is, has not revealed to us all the phenomena which take place in it. (p. 18)

It is interesting to speculate on whether this case of Ménière's may be the
first clinical description of benign paroxysmal positional vertigo (BPPV). The
brief sudden spells of vertigo triggered by getting in or out of bed are typical of
the disorder. Clearly, the young man had more than just positional vertigo, but
people with BPPV can have other symptoms of inner ear disease. Unfortunately,
Ménière did not provide enough information to be certain of the diagnosis.

Even more interesting is whether his patient had what has subsequently
become known as Ménière's disease. The modem diagnostic criteria for Ménière's
disease include spontaneous attacks of vertigo, tinnitus, and hearing loss. The
key to the diagnosis is worsening hearing loss during the attack of vertigo. This
young man had spontaneous vertigo followed by tinnitus and fluctuating hearing loss, but it is unclear whether they occurred together. When the hearing
symptoms began, they involved both ears. The hearing loss with Ménière's disease invariably begins in one ear and remains so for years, and only a small per-
centage of patients go on to develop involvement of both ears after many years.

Complicating matters further, Ménière (1861b) noted that people with
migraine often had symptoms similar to those of the young man (as translated in
Atkinson, 1961): "I do not hesitate to regard these migraines as dependent upon
a lesion of the inner ear; they are accompanied by noises, by vertigo, by gradual
diminution of hearing, and most often their deafness resists all methods of treatment" (p. 21). We now know that migraine can mimic Ménière's disease and
probably cause Ménière's disease in a small subset of people. There is a signifi-
cantly higher incidence of migraine in people with Ménière's disease compared
to people without Ménière's disease. Ménière, who had migraine headaches
himself, went on to point out that migraine is very common, so it should be relatively easy for future investigators to clarify the association between migraine
and inner ear symptoms. Ménière was overoptimistic, however, because there is
still controversy regarding the mechanism of inner ear symptoms with migraine.

Ménière seemed frustrated in his efforts to obtain an exact history from his
young patient (Ménière, 1861b). He noted (as translated in Atkinson, 1961),

> With some patients more observant of what happens to them I have
> found it possible by means of very precise questioning to establish that
> the vertigo, the collapse, the sudden fall, the vomiting, have been pre-
> ceded by noises in the ears. (p. 17)

He then described other cases with the more classical symptom complex of
modem-day Ménière's disease. Ménière was particularly fond of describing

physician patients because he believed that they were more observant of their symptoms. This may be true in some cases, but in my experience physicians are often the worst historians because they interpret rather than describe their symptoms.

More Evidence That Vertigo Can Originate from the Inner Ear

Ménière went on to provide other arguments that vertigo could result from damage to the inner ears. In the course of his practice at the Deaf-Mute Institute, he had seen numerous patients who developed vertigo and hearing loss after a foreign object such as a tree branch entered the ear canal. When he examined some of these cases soon after the injury, there was no evidence of brain damage yet they suffered from a "cerebral symptom"—vertigo. He concluded that the objects penetrated the inner ear, causing vertigo and hearing loss.

Possibly the most convincing argument that vertigo could originate from damage to the inner ear was his report of the autopsy findings in a young girl who experienced sudden hearing loss and acute vertigo (Ménière, 1861b; as translated in Atkinson, 1961):

> A girl who having journeyed by night in winter on the box seat of a coach during the time of her catemania became as a result of the severe cold completely and suddenly deaf. Admitted to the service of M. Chomel, she presented as principal symptom continuous vertigo, least effort at movement caused vomiting and death supervened on the fifth day. (p. 18)

At autopsy, Ménière found that the brain and spinal cord were completely normal but, when examining the child's inner ear, he noted a red plastic material, a bloody exudate, filling the semicircular canals but not the cochlea (the hearing part of the inner ear). On the basis of this single case, he established an essential correlation between vertigo and the inner ear. In retrospect, this was likely a case of acute leukemia with hemorrhage into the inner ear. It provided convincing evidence that damage to the semicircular canals of the inner ear causes vertigo, but it also led to a great deal of controversy.

Inconsistencies in Ménière's Description of the Young Girl with Vertigo

More than a decade before his seminal paper, Ménière translated a German book on diseases of the ear by Kramer (1848) with his own personal notes and additions. He described the same circumstances of the young girl travel-ing at night in an open carriage but reported only that she had been stricken with complete and absolute deafness in the space of a few hours. When he examined the temporal bones (part of the skull that contains the inner ear), he found a plastic, reddish lymph throughout the inner ear that appeared to be the result of an exudation from all the membranous surfaces lining the inner ear. He made no mention of vertigo in this initial report, and he clearly stated that the reddish fluid bathed the entire inner ear. Apparently, he had not for-mulated his theory on the association between vertigo and the inner ear at the time of this earlier report. Assuming he thought the vertigo was of cerebral origin, it was not worth noting. It is more difficult to understand, however, the discrepancy between the report of selective involvement of the semicir-cular canals in his paper of 1861 and the report of generalized involvement of the inner ear in the report of 1848. "Was Ménière's first account careless, was his memory faulty, or did his desire to reinforce his conviction that the dam-age in the case he was describing was in the semicircular canals lead him to stretch the evidence?" asked noted Ménière historian Miles Atkinson (1961). Atkinson concluded,

> Even if the last is the explanation—and I confess it is one which seems most plausible, it is no damning criticism of Ménière. Many an honest man has done the same thing before and since. It is a human failing, to which even the integrity of the scientist is not always immune, to try to fit facts into a favored pattern, even if they are not of exactly the right shape. It is one aspect of what, in the parlance of the day, is called wish-ful thinking. (pp. 67–68)

In other words, science is not always orderly and precise because human beings by nature are not always orderly and precise.

An unexpected result of Ménière's description of the young girl's autopsy was its effect on subsequent debate regarding the cause of Ménière's disease. As discussed later (see Chapter 13), in 1938 English and Japanese researchers found hydrops (swelling) of the inner ear in autopsy specimens from patients who had the typical symptoms of Ménière's disease. However, because of Ménière's description of the young girl's autopsy in his classical paper, the con-cept that Ménière's disease was caused by hemorrhage into the inner ear per-sisted into the 1950s. Obviously, Ménière was not suggesting that his patients with episodic vertigo, tinnitus, and fluctuating hearing loss had the same dis-ease as the young girl with sudden deafness and vertigo. He was simply making the point that vertigo and hearing loss commonly occur together with inner ear disease.

Treatments for Vertigo in the Mid-19th Century

Ménière provided a remarkably detailed description of the range of treatments used at that time for patients with vertigo (Ménière, 1861b). He described a physician who consulted him because of the classical symptom triad of Ménière's disease (vertigo, tinnitus, and hearing loss). This physician had tried just about everything available prior to consulting Ménière. He started with sulfite of quinine, but this drug only produced louder head noises and temporary deafness, well-known side effects of quinine. Ménière noted (as translated in Atkinson, 1961),

> Supposing a dyspepsia was the origin of his vertigo and vomiting, our colleague made use of all the medications vaunted in such cases— tonics, debilitants, iron compounds, bitters, charged waters, ice within and without then irritant applications, blistering fluids on the epigastrium, rubefacient lotions, Croton oil, antimonial ointment—all of these without result. Believing then that the affectation was a cerebral one, he had himself bled often and copiously. He put numbers of leeches to the temples and behind the ears, but the general debility produced by this spoliation appeared to increase the illness and from then on this physician assumed that he was suffering from a cachectic state, the result of certain youthful errors. Thereupon, iodide of potassium was taken regularly in large doses and for several months, 2 grams and more of this salt were absorbed every day. (p. 30)

Despite all of these measures, the physician's symptoms of vertigo, tinnitus, and deafness continued, and he then began to consider that his symptoms were originating from the inner ear. With this in mind, he had a large seton placed in the nape of his neck. A seton is a large curved needle threaded with string soaked in strong salt solution. When the string was left in place for a few days, it produced suppuration that was supposed to draw off the inflammation. When this was not successful, he had moxas-cotton in the shape of a cone impregnated with potassium chlorate placed on the skin behind the ear and then lit. The resulting burn drew off the bad humors, inflammation, or whatever was causing the trouble. When this was not effective, he went on to sulfur waters and Turkish baths. Ménière (1861b) noted (as translated in Atkinson, 1961),

> He used and abused everything which could be taken no matter in what form. The disease did not yield even to electricity, not even to ether instilled into the ears so that the patient at the end of his resources decided at least to have recourse to physicians who concerned

themselves more particularly with affectations of the auditory apparatus. He consulted them all, submitted himself patiently to their pre-
scriptions and finished by understanding that his deafness, as I had
conceived it my duty to tell him at our very first interview, was not one
of those where art could usefully intervene. He is fully convinced of it
today, and had resigned himself to it, seeking to do the best of the little
hearing which remains to him. (p. 31)

Ménière's Comments Trigger Heated Debate

Ménière's paper was politely shelved by appointing a commission to consider and report on the work (a common policy for papers presented at the
Academy). However, in the same auditorium at the Academy of Medicine
meeting the following week, M. Armand Trousseau, physician-in-chief of
the Hôtel-Dieu, read a paper titled "Concerning Apoplectiform Cerebral
Congestion in Its Relation to Epilepsy" (Trousseau, 1861). In this paper,
Trousseau questioned the usefulness of such a diagnosis as apoplectiform
cerebral congestion, noting that it undoubtedly consists of many different
individual disorders, each of which should be considered as a separate diagnosis. As an example, he cited Ménière's paper from the previous week and the
vertigo syndrome that Ménière described. Because Trousseau was a member
of the Academy and because of his high stature, a lively discussion followed
and continued for the next 6 weeks (Atkinson, 1961). Although Ménière was
disbarred from entering into this discussion himself, he was keenly interested
in Trousseau's opinions, and he immediately wrote a critical report that was
published in the *Gazette Medicale* on January 26, 1861 (Ménière, 1861c; as
translated in Atkinson, 1961). He commented on the complexity of the condition of apoplectic cerebral congestion and on the injudicious nature of the
conventional treatment. He wanted to "open the eyes of practitioners who are
a little too inclined to practice bleeding from the arm on some of the alleged
apoplectics, to put leeches on the neck or on the buttocks of people who were
in fact anemic" (p. 36). Bleeding a patient with anemia may seem ludicrous,
but it was a common practice at that time. Of course, if the people were not
anemic at the start of treatment, they were anemic after a month or two of
bleeding therapy. Ménière wrote a strenuous defense of Trousseau and his
suggestion that apoplectiform cerebral congestion consisted of many different disorders, and he expressed hope that the paper would stimulate further
discussion.

The comments of Ménière and Trousseau must have created quite a storm
in the Parisian medical community. They were questioning ingrained principles

with foundations in the teachings of the great Greek physicians Hippocrates and Galen. As noted previously, although scientific methodology was beginning to affect medical thinking, it had little effect on the average medical practitioner in the mid-19th century. The severity of the criticism leveled against Ménière and Trousseau is obvious from reading Ménière's response to their detractors. Ménière (1861c; as translated in Atkinson, 1961) pleaded that

> one must allow to each the right to express himself as best he may, above all when the words which he uses express his thought and make no pretense to obtrude upon anybody. Anyhow, to what end lead quarrels about words? Is there anything more empty, more useless and at the same time more irritating? (p. 43)

He went on to attempt to defend Trousseau, who apparently was taking the brunt of the criticism, arguing that if a physician has the patient's interest at heart he will be willing to consider new ideas and look for new answers: "Let us give thanks to seeking spirits, to those with initiative, who raise questions of interest, stimulate active researches, provoke opposition, because, in a word, science gains and humanity applauds" (p. 43).

After several weeks of heated debate that included personal attacks, Trousseau had had enough and called off the debate at the Academy. Although Ménière was obviously disillusioned, he continued to collect and report additional cases with vertigo and hearing loss that he published in the *Gazette Medicale* in February, April, and June of 1861 (Ménière, 1861d, 1861e, 1861f). He wrote right up until the day before his unexpected death on February 7, 1862, due to influenza pneumonia.

References

Ackerknecht EH, Vallois HV. *Franz Joseph Gall, Inventor of Phrenology and His Collection*. Transl by St Leon C, Department of History of Medicine, University of Wisconsin Medical School, Madison, Wisconsin, 1956.

Atkinson M. Ménière's original papers. *Acta Otolaryngol (Stockh)* [Suppl] 1961;162:1–78.

Baloh RW. Prosper Meniere and his disease. *Arch Neurol* 2001;58:1151–1156.

Canalis RF, Mira E, Bonandrini L, Hinojosa R. Antonio Scarpa and the discovery of the membranous inner ear. *Otol Neurotol* 2001;22:105–112.

Changeux J-P. *Neuronal Man: The Biology of Mind*. Transl by Garey L, Princeton, NJ: Princeton University Press, 1985.

Flourens P. Recherches expérimentales sur les propriétés et les functions du système nerveux dans les animaux vertébrés. Paris: Crevot, 1842.

Kramer W. *Traité des maladies de l'oreille*. Transl by P. Ménière. Paris: Germer-Bailliere, 1848.

Ménière P. Sur une forme de surdite grave dependant d'une lesion de l'oreille interne. *Gaz Méd Paris* 1861a;16:29.

Ménière P. Mémoire sur des lésions de l'oreille interne donnant lieu à des symptômes de congestion cérébrale apoplectiforme. *Gaz Méd Paris* 1861b;16:597–601.

Ménière P. Académie de Médecine: Congestions cérébrales apoplectiforme: M. Trousseau. Discussion: MM. Bouillaud, Piorry, Tardieu, Durand-Fardel. *Gaz Med Paris* 1861c;16:55–57.

Ménière P. Maladies de l'oreille interne offrant les symptômes de la congestion cérébrale apoplectiforme. *Gaz Med Paris* 1861d;16:88–89.

Ménière P. Nouveaux documents relatifs aux lesions de l'oreille interne caractérisées par des symptomes de congestion cerebrale apoplectiforme. *Gaz Méd Paris* 1861e;16:239–240.

Ménière P. Observations de maladies de l'oreille interne caracterisees par des symptômes de congestion cerebrale apoplectiforme. *Gaz Med Paris* 1861f;16:379–380.

Pappas DG. Otology through the ages. *Otolaryngol Head Neck Surg* 1996;114:173–196.

Pearce JMS. Marie-Jean-Pierre Flourens (1794–1867) and cortical localization. *Eur Neurol* 2009;61:1–8.

Scarpa A. *Anatomicae disquisitions de auditu et olfacta*. Pavia, Italy: Pietro Galleati, 1789.

Talbott JH. *A Biographical History of Medicine: Excerpts and Essays on the Men and Their Work*. New York: Grune & Stratton, 1970.

Trousseau A. De la congestion cérébrale apoplectiforme, dans ses rapports avec épilepsie. *Gaz Méd Paris* 1861;16:51.

3

Ménière, a Man of Many Interests

Prosper Ménière was born on June 18, 1799, in Angers, France, the same year that Napoleon Bonaparte came to power (Atkinson, 1961). He was the third of four children born to a prosperous merchant in this city in western France noted for its wineries, nurseries, and market gardens. Ménière received an excellent education in the classics, and he maintained his scholarly interest in the classics throughout his life. The beautiful nurseries and gardens of Angers stimulated Ménière's interest in botany, which he also maintained throughout his life. He became a member of the local botany society while he was a teenager, and in later years he was elected vice president. Ménière went on to join the Botanical Society of France, of which he also was elected vice president.

Ménière witnessed remarkable political upheaval during his lifetime. He grew up in the First Empire, the "glory years," benefiting from Napoleon's strong support of education in the arts and humanities. He entered secondary school at age 13 years in 1812, the year of Napoleon's retreat from Moscow. He was studying the classics in 1815 during the time of Napoleon's return from exile, his defeat by Wellington at Waterloo, and his final exile to the island of St. Helena. Ménière was a young physician at the Hôtel-Dieu of Paris in 1830, where he cared for hundreds of injured citizens during the Battle of the Barricades, part of France's so-called "second revolution." Finally, Ménière lived the last 10 years of his life in the Second Empire, which began in 1852 when Napoleon's nephew Prince Louis Napoleon replaced the "citizen king" Louis-Philippe.

Ménière's Academic Career

Ménière completed 3 years at the Preparatory School of Medicine at the University of Angers before moving to Paris in 1819 to complete his medical studies. He received his doctorate of medicine in 1828 and was appointed as an aide in the clinic of the famous surgeon Baron Dupuytren in the Hôtel-Dieu.

The Hôtel-Dieu of Paris was founded in approximately 652 by St. Landrey, the 28th bishop of Paris (Talbott, 1970). Located next to Notre-Dame, it was the first hospital in Paris and is the oldest hospital in the world still operating (Figure 3.1). The medieval Hôtel-Dieu of Paris was known for its enormous rooms with massive beds holding four to six patients. There was a wealth of clinical teaching material, providing Ménière with excellent clinical training. During the 3 days of the Battle of the Barricades mentioned previously, 204 casualties were admitted to the Hôtel-Dieu on July 29, 1830, while Ménière was working. One can imagine the massive rooms of the Hôtel-Dieu overflowing with wounded citizens and the sisters and physicians scurrying about caring for them.

In 1833, Ménière was appointed chief of the clinic of Auguste-Francois Chomel, Professor of Medicine and noted academician. This was really the beginning of Ménière's academic career, and there is little doubt that Ménière's ultimate goal was to become a professor at the Hôtel-Dieu (Atkinson, 1961). In 1835, Ménière was sent by the government to the department of Aude and of the Haute Garonne to help quell an epidemic of cholera. For his efforts, he was made a Chevalier of the Legion of Honor. Despite his accomplishments, however, Ménière did not receive the appointment he desired at the Hôtel-Dieu. On two separate occasions, he was considered first in line for a professorship, but on both occasions the position was given to a lesser qualified candidate, presumably for political reasons.

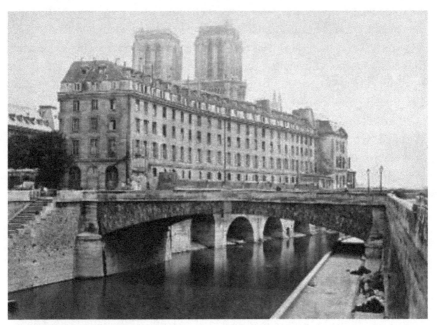

Figure 3.1 HÔTEL-DIEU DE PARIS IN THE MID-19TH CENTURY. Source: Photographed by Charles Marville in approximately 1865.

The year 1838 marked a turning point in Ménière's life. Jean Marie Gaspar Itard, one of the founding fathers of otology and a pioneer in the education of the deaf, died while he was serving as director of the Imperial Institute for Deaf-Mutes in Paris. Even though he had no formal training in otology, Ménière was offered the post as director and devoted the remainder of his life caring for and writing about "his poor deaf-mutes" (Pappas and McGuinn, 1993).

Ménière Balances Academic, Patient, and Family Activities

In his day-to-day work at the Deaf-Mute Institute, Ménière experienced the usual trials and tribulations of academic medicine: the fatiguing work of patient care balanced with the need to publish ("publish or perish"). From the many letters that Ménière wrote to friends and relatives, it is clear that he had mixed feelings about his patient responsibilities (Pappas and McGuinn, 1993). He enjoyed talking to patients and taking a careful history. He obviously took great joy in making the correct diagnosis and being able to provide the patients with appropriate treatment. On the other hand, he frequently complained about the heavy workload. He complained about being inundated with consultations from morning to late afternoon so that his head was "in a hash." He described a typical Sunday activity in which he visited two infirmaries, passed in review all of the students gathered in the great gallery, visited a sick woman in Rue de Tournay, and then, after returning home, found another batch of patients whom he was obliged to examine. On one occasion, he wrote how he detested returning to Paris after a holiday because "the patients would be waiting for me there in droves." In a letter dated August 26, 1853, he tersely summarized how draining of energy it could be after a full day of seeing patients: He wrote, "I saw more than 20 patients, I worked, I talked, and I found the time short until evening."

Ménière was constantly concerned about finding quality time to write because he was so tired from his patient work. Despite this concern, he was a prolific writer. He maintained his long-standing interest in botany, writing several papers on orchids. He wrote on the classics, including a treatise on the medical knowledge of the classical Latin poets. He wrote critical essays, obituaries, and historical reviews. Miles Atkinson (1961) noted, "Ménière was an enthusiastic letter writer, sending a long letter every week to a favorite niece, writing to his friend Lachese in Angers and to others" (p. 73). His first medical monograph, titled *Memoire sur la grossesse interstitielle*, was published in 1826. His landmark publication on treatment of deaf-mutes, *De la guerison de la surdimutite et de l'education des sourds-muets*, was published in 1853. As noted previously, his famous paper on the inner ear and vertigo was published in the *Gazette*

Medicale in September 1861. His final monograph, *Ciceron medecin*, was published in 1862 just before his death.

The way that Ménière went about educating himself on the anatomy, physiology, and pathology of the ear after his appointment to head the Deaf-Mute Institute in 1838 provides insight to his analytic approach. He read the standard French texts available on inner ear diseases, including Itard's two-volume work titled *Treatment of Diseases of the Ear*. He then went on to translate the German textbook on ear diseases by Kramer because he wanted to broaden his overall knowledge on the subject. He was not satisfied with a simple translation of Kramer's work, however, and maintained a running dialogue correcting Kramer whenever he disagreed with him and adding his own personal observations whenever he though them appropriate (Kramer, 1848). As noted previously, it was in this context that he mentioned the history and autopsy results of the young girl who had the sudden onset of vertigo and hearing loss.

Despite Ménière's many academic accomplishments, all indications are that he remained humble (Pappas and McGuinn, 1993). When writing to a colleague, who was interested in putting together a collection of his works, Ménière stated, "Who knows if among this jumble there will one day be manifested two good lines to preserve? One can say, I believe, that immortality is not the lot of little books, nor does one attain posterity with great baggage" (p. 322). Regarding his feelings toward fame and recognition from his work, Ménière wrote,

> I obey my instincts in writing these things which pass through my head;
> I attach little importance to fame, and even less to people in general.
> I find that the world does not vaunt the efforts which one takes to
> please it. (p. 322)

One wonders whether these cynical comments arose from a rejection of one of his written products. Most writers have had these sentiments at some time or another.

Ménière relied on Divine Providence (as quoted in Pappas and McGuinn, 1993): "I like to allow Providence to speak for me. I do not wish to influence it. . . . Do we know what best befits us? Is it not necessary to be content with our lot, whatever it be?" (p. 323). Although Ménière was well known and popular in the Parisian medical community, he had received several setbacks, including his failure to receive the professorship at the Hôtel-Dieu and his failure to be elected to the Imperial Academy of Medicine. There apparently was political intrigue involved in both of these academic failures, but Ménière took them philosophically. "He knew that justice was not of this world, and that to delude himself, man relies on a mirage of words," wrote the Swiss otologist Charles Albert Fiessinger (1903, p. 9). Ménière had a pessimistic view of his contributions to posterity (as quoted in Pappas and McGuinn, 1993):

> I am certain that the best works have been burned, that the sweetest verses have never been printed, that what is more charming in human thought lied buried in these catacombs, where modesty so willingly conceals itself; whereas the shameless, the impertinent, the preeminent show off with insolence in the sun of publicity without any right to do so. (p. 322)

He had the right degree of cynicism to flourish in our modern society.

Ménière's Everyday Life

There is relatively little information about Ménière's family life in his extensive writings. In the same year that he became director of the Deaf-Mute Institute, he married Mlle. Becquerel, the daughter of a professor at the Paris Botanical Garden (Pappas and McGuinn, 1993). His wife came from a distinguished scientific family that included Henri Becquerel, who received the Nobel Prize in 1903 for the discovery of radioactivity. Their only son Emil became an otologist like his father and ultimately held the same position as his father at the Institute for Deaf-Mutes. Ménière and his wife had a very active social schedule, attending parties, the opera, the theater, and often dining out. He gave some hint of how he felt about some of these social occasions when he noted that his wife was complaining of idleness and that they were going to be visiting the home of friends that Sunday for an evening of concert and dance—"a lengthy boredom for me, for there is a crowd of people I do not like. But all in all, one must resign oneself to it, meet one's obligations as a married man, and yawn officially" (as quoted in Pappas and McGuinn, 1993, p. 325). Atkinson (1961) speculated that the reason we know so little about Ménière's personal life is that his son Emil, who edited and published his father's letters after his death, probably edited out most of the family references.

With Ménière's busy schedule of seeing patients and writing, there were two things that he feared more than anything else—colds and migraine headaches (Pappas and McGuinn, 1993). He was predisposed to catching colds that he obviously dreaded. In one of his letters, he noted that an upholsterer had come to lay a new carpet to protect him from his dreaded colds. In another, he complained about how terribly cold it was in Paris that winter but so far he had not gotten one of his usual colds (as quoted in Pappas and McGuinn, 1993):

> I am looking after myself well and taking many precautions. I do not wish to yield beneath the weight of the years, beneath the attacks of this stinging cold weather. I am increasing my efforts to counterbalance these burning enemies, these illnesses: May heaven cause me to escape their embraces! (p. 322)

The only thing that he dreaded more than a cold was one of his migraine headaches. In a letter to his niece, he described how a migraine headache came on in the evening, forcing him to cancel a visit to the opera. He slept for 12 hours, and the next morning he felt well again only to have the headache overtake him in the late morning (as quoted in Pappas and McGuinn, 1993):

> I wish to receive my patients; I spoke, I wrote—all to the great detriment of my brain, I assure you. What to do for this cruel pain? I have drunk torrents of tea, I have dieted; I close my eyes, I remain quiet. . . . I am having 15 people to dinner. I must do what I must to be agreeable, to converse with this numerous society. (pp. 322–323)

Ménière's Role in French Society

In the years that he served as director of the Deaf-Mute Institute, Ménière socialized with some of the most prominent members of mid-19th-century France. Despite his claims to the contrary, Ménière was probably as well known a figure in society as he was a physician (Atkinson, 1961). He was particularly close to theater critic Jules Gabriel Janin. He mentions Janin repeatedly in his letters, and they spent a great deal of time together socially. In one letter, he noted that Janin was unable to go to the theater because of gout, so Ménière attended the theater and provided Janin with the details to write his critical review. Ménière was particularly fond of Italian opera, frequently using the phrase "I must go to the Italians." He apparently felt guilty balancing his busy social and work schedule. In a letter to his niece, he tried to defend his social life (as quoted in Pappas and McGuinn, 1993):

> You scold me, my child, for my long evenings, for my plays, for a very worldly life, but can I behave otherwise? I went yesterday to the Italians for Lucia, from which I returned enchanted. I refuse to go to the comic opera this evening for a premiere performance—see what strength I have. (p. 325)

Ménière had an interesting relationship with the great French novelist Honore Balzac. They initially were close friends, and Balzac used Ménière as an intern at the Hôtel-Dieu in his novel, *Peau de chagrin*. At approximately that time, Ménière's close friend Janin angered Balzac with one of his reviews, and a major feud developed between the two literary giants. In a letter dated June 1858, Ménière noted that he had to stop seeing Balzac once Balzac became aware of his connection with Janin (Fiessinger, 1903). He lamented the fact that the two men never had the least relationship yet they despised each other. To illustrate his point, Fiessinger quoted Ménière's description of an outburst by Balzac:

> I will have an immense fortune, millions to eclipse Rothschild, I will have a palace of marble and gold, I will receive the most noble people, I will give sumptuous dinners, magnificent concerts, everyone will come to my house, Janin alone will not come, and will burst with spite for it! (pp. 10–11)

In later editions of *Peau de chagrin*, Balzac changed the name of the Ménière character, presumably because of his continuing feud with Janin.

All in all, Ménière was a complex man with many different interests and many talents. As he was well aware, fame is fleeting, and it is impossible to predict how one will be judged by posterity. Ménière would have been the last to predict that his paper presented before the Imperial Academy of Medicine in January 1861 would lead to a type of immortality. The disease he described established his name in perpetuity.

References

Atkinson M. Ménière's original papers. *Acta Otolaryngol (Stockh)* [Suppl] 1961;162:1–78.

Fiessinger CA. *Biographie du docteur Prosper Ménière, professeur agrégé à l'École de Médecine, médecin en chef des Sourds-Muets, chevalier de la Légion d'Honneur, 1799–1862. Journal de docteur Prosper Meniere, publié par son fils le Dr. E. M Ménière.* Paris: Plon-Nourrit, 1903.

Kramer W. *Traité des maladies de l'oreille.* Transl P. Méniere. Paris: Germer-Bailliere, 1848.

Ménière P. Mémoire sur des lésions de l'oreille interne donnant lieu à des symptômes de congestion cérébrale apoplectiforme. *Gaz Méd Paris* 1861;16:597–601.

Pappas DG, McGuinn MG. Unpublished letters from Prosper Ménière: A personal silhouette. *Am J Otol* 1993;14:318–325.

Talbott JH. *A Biographical History of Medicine: Excerpts and Essays on the Men and Their Work.* New York: Grune & Stratton, 1970.

JOSEF BREUER (1842–1925)

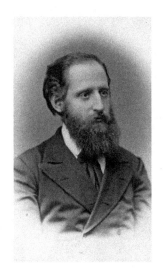

Josef Breuer was 19 years old in the second year of medical school at the University of Vienna when Ménière presented his famous paper before the Academy of Medicine in Paris in 1861. Breuer would go on to discover the neural basis for the self-regulation of respiration (the Hering–Breuer reflex); describe how the balance part of the inner ear (the vestibular system) works; and, along with Sigmund Freud, develop the field of psychoanalysis. His body of work on the physiology of the vestibular system is probably greater than that of any other single investigator. With the exception of only a few minor details, his findings published more than 150 years ago are still considered valid by modern-day researchers. Even more remarkable is the fact that all of his work on the inner ear was conducted while he was maintaining a busy private practice. He worked in a few small rooms at home in the evenings and during the night using equipment purchased from the fees of his medical practice.

Breuer Discovers How the Balance Portion of the Inner Ear Works

Breuer presented his initial work on the inner ear in the form of a preliminary communication to the session of the Imperial Society of Physicians in Vienna on November 14, 1873, published in the journal of the Society on November 20, 1873 (Breuer, 1873); he also published a more detailed paper in the medical yearbook of the Society of Physicians in 1874 (Breuer,1874). His basic premise was that the semicircular canals sense angular movement of the head by movement of the fluid (endolymph) within them. The endolymph moves relative to the walls of the canals because of its inertia. Because the three semicircular canals are approximately at right angles to each other, the canals sense movement in all possible planes. Within each semicircular canal there is a bulbous enlargement called the ampulla where the sensory receptor, the crista, is located (Figure 4.1; see also Figure 1.1). In dissecting the semicircular canals of pigeons, he noted nerve endings contacting cells at the base of the ampulla and microscopic hairs extending from the top of the cells into a gelatinous bulb (called the cupula). He hypothesized that movement of the endolymph fluid triggered by angular head movements bent the tiny hairs, activating the nerve endings at the base of the hair cells. The nerves in turn passed on signals reflecting the direction and magnitude of hair deflection to the central nervous system.

Breuer was familiar with the work of the German physiologist Goltz (1870), who had concluded that the semicircular canals were sense organs for equilibrium of the head, but he disagreed with Goltz's interpretation that the mechanism of the sensory transduction is due to hydrostatic pressure of the endolymph on the membranous semicircular canals. Breuer argued that Goltz's theory was impossible on physical grounds because a closed ring filled with fluid would not exhibit fluctuations of internal pressure according to the spatial position of the system. He argued that rotation of such a ring in its own plane would cause the endolymph to be displaced relative to the ring, and that the endolymph flow would cease after a certain period of time as a result of friction at the walls. To

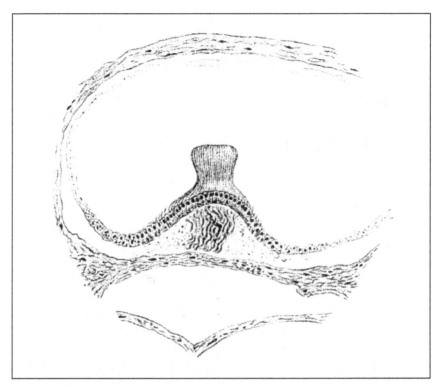

Figure 4.1 Breuer's drawing of a cross section of the horizontal semicircular ampulla from a pigeon. One can see the cilia of the hair cells protruding into the cupula and the afferent nerve innervating the hair cells. The cupula does not span the ampulla due to postmortem shrinkage. Source: From Breuer J. Studien über den Vestibularapparat. *S Ber Akad Wiss Wien math-naturw K1* 1903;112:315–394.

explain how this movement of endolymph within the semicircular canal could lead to activation of nerve terminals, Breuer suggested an analogy with the lateral line organs in fish. These primitive forerunners of the semicircular canals sense movements in the water by bending of the receptor. Interestingly, many years later, it would be the detailed measurement of the nerve firing from the lateral line organs of fish that would provide more detailed understanding of how the sensory transduction process in the inner ear works (Hoagland, 1933; Löwenstein and Sand, 1936).

In his study of pigeons, Breuer noted that the entire head oscillated with slow and quick back-and-forth movements in response to rotating the animal in the plane of one of the semicircular canals, a phenomenon that he called "nystagmus of the head." He went on to suggest that Flourens' finding of head and body movements in pigeons that occurred after a semicircular canal was damaged was the same phenomenon (Flourens, 1842). In other words, the head and body movements observed by Flourens represented reflexive movements resulting from damage to the semicircular canal. He suggested and later carried out more detailed experiments on pigeons that conclusively proved this theory.

Eye Movements and the Semicircular Canals

Breuer also performed a series of experiments in human subjects, including himself, rotating in the plane of a pair of semicircular canals on a rotating platform. Unlike pigeons, humans only had eye nystagmus, not head nystagmus. The nystagmus had slow and fast phases that occurred in the plane of rotation. The slow-phase eye movement was equal in magnitude and opposite in direction to the head movement (i.e., compensatory) so that the eyes would automatically stay fixed on an object of interest. The fast-phase eye movements simply kept the eyes near the center of the orbits so that they did not become pinned to one side. The semicircular canals only sensed angular acceleration because the nystagmus began with the onset of rotation and gradually decayed once a constant velocity was reached. The slow and fast phases of the nystagmus reversed direction on stopping the rotation (deacceleration), and again the nystagmus gradually decayed. He convinced himself that these ocular oscillations were purely reflex in nature because they occurred even when he rotated blind subjects. Although others including Purkinje, the famous Czech physiologist (Grüsser, 1984), had previously observed nystagmus associated with rotation of normal human subjects, Breuer was the first to explain the compensatory nature of the eye movement and its direct relationship to stimulating the semicircular canals. The function of these reflexive compensatory eye movements is to keep vision stable during head movements (the so-called vestibulo-ocular reflexes). A major symptom of people who have lost these reflexes due to damage to the semicircular canals or vestibular nerves is oscillopsia, the sense that objects are moving whenever the head is moving. Such people can have difficulty reading even when they are still because tiny movements of the head associated with the heart beating can lead to tiny eye movements that diminish visual acuity.

The Gravity-Sensing Otolith Organs

In his initial formulation on how the semicircular canals work, Breuer relied on a combination of a review of the work of other contemporary investigators and his own personal observations from experiments in pigeons and human subjects. He went on to emphasize that in addition to the semicircular canals, the inner ear contains sensory receptors for linear acceleration including gravity. These linear accelerometers were necessary to compliment the angular accelerometers in the semicircular canals to provide the brain with a complete set of orienting signals. These organs, called the macules or otolith organs, were also critical for perceiving the static position of the head—the degree of head tilt.

Evolutionary Development of the Inner Ear

All living organisms have the ability to orient with respect to gravity—to determine up from down. Even the most basic single-cell forms of life, such as bacteria and algae, detect the pull of gravity by differences in density at different parts of the cell. A specialized organ to sense gravity is already seen in primitive animals such as the jellyfish, which appeared more than 600 million years ago on the evolutionary timescale. The jellyfish has a pouch filled with seawater containing tiny stones, "liths," whose density is much greater than that of the surrounding fluid (Figure 4.2). Due to gravity, these tiny stones rest their weight on specialized sensory cells (hair cells) in the walls of the pouch, allowing the animals to regulate their position in space.

The primitive gravity-sensing organ, the otolith (ear stone) organ or statocyst, is the forerunner of the inner ear of animals higher up on the evolutionary

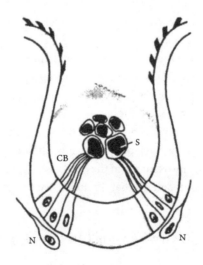

Figure 4.2 STATOCYST OF A JELLYFISH. A ciliary bundle (CB) from hair cells supports the extracellular statoliths (S). Nerve cells (N) at the base monitor the activity of the hair cells and carry the information to the animal's nervous system to generate orienting postural reflexes. Source: From Budelmann BU. Morphological diversity of equilibrium receptor systems in aquatic invertebrates. In: Atema J, et al. (eds). *Sensory Biology of Aquatic Animals.* Springer-Verlag, New York, 1988.

scale. The statocyst in mollusks (e.g., octopuses) has both a static receptor (the macule) and a kinetic receptor (the crista). Both receptors are located in a common cavity. The pouch previously open to the outside is closed and filled with fluid (endolymph) secreted by cells in the wall of the cyst. The development of a kinetic receptor marks the appearance of kinetic reflexes such as the vestibulo-ocular reflex and nystagmus. The macule of the octopus consists of a rounded plate of mechanosensory cells covered by a single large statolith, whereas the crista consists of a narrow strip of mechanosensory cells winding around the inside of the cyst overlayed by a sail-like cupula that is deflected during rotational movements of the animal by flow of endolymph relative to the cyst wall. Each organ relies on the basic feature of mechanosensory cells, hair cells, acting as force transducers for linear and angular acceleration.

Surviving primitive fish illustrate the phylogenetic development of the vestibular part of the inner ear. The inner ear of the hagfish has a single circular tube interrupted by two bulbous enlargements, the ampullae, each containing a primitive crista with overlying cupula. A common macule, the forerunner of the utricular and saccular macules, lies in an intercommunicating channel between the ampullae. In the lamprey, the channel becomes a bilobulated sac containing separate utricular and saccular macules.

Primitive auditory organs, the lagenar macule and the basilar papilla, first appear in the saccule once the membranous sac is divided into two cavities. In birds, the basilar papilla becomes a long, uncoiled organ, the predecessor of the coiled cochlea of mammals. All mammals have the same basic inner ear structure that includes three semicircular canals—the utricle, the saccule, and the cochlea.

Mach and His Psychophysical Experiments

A week before Breuer submitted his material to the Imperial Society of Physicians, Ernst Mach, a professor of physics in Prague, sent a paper with similar findings and conclusions to the Vienna Academy of Sciences (Mach, 1873). Mach and Breuer arrived at their theories completely independently based on different experiences and different kinds of information. Mach, like Breuer, had multiple interests and made major contributions in many different fields (Blackmore, 1972). He is probably best known for his work in the area of fluid mechanics, in which his name is used as the unit for the speed of sound. His knowledge in psychophysics and fluid dynamics provided an ideal background for his study of inner ear function in humans. Mach described how he became interested in the subject (as quoted in Blackmore, 1972): "On rounding a railway curve once, I accidentally observed a striking apparent inclination of the houses and trees" (p. 51). Being a physicist, Mach was well aware of the linear acceleration

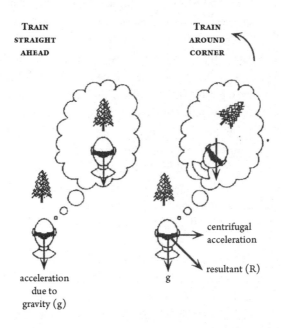

Figure 4.3 ILLUSION OF TILT EXPERIENCED BY MACH ON A TRAIN GOING AROUND A CORNER. The otolith organs in the inner ear sense the resultant (R) of the outward centrifugal acceleration and the downward acceleration due to gravity (g) and send this signal on to the brain. The brain interprets R as the direction of gravity (up and down), leading to the illusion of tilt.

associated with a centrifugal movement and how this vector would summate with the acceleration vector due to gravity producing a resultant vector R, the new perceived vertical (Figure 4.3). He convinced himself that the sensors for linear acceleration are located in the head because the illusion of tilt was unaffected by body movement as long as the head remained still. Conversely, head movements with the body still altered the perception of tilt.

To prove his theory that the inner ear was the organ responsible for sensing linear and angular acceleration, Mach built a rotating device designed so that it could rotate experimental subjects about multiple axes (Figure 4.4). The chair on which the subject sat could be moved from the center of rotation so that a centrifugal force was produced. To control visual stimuli, he covered the rotating chair with a paper box, with a pointer inside the box connected to a similar pointer outside that the person used to indicate the subjective vertical. Unlike Breuer, Mach focused on the subjective sensation of rotation rather than the reflexive eye movements (nystagmus) induced by rotation. With his rotational device, he was able to clearly show that receptors in the head sensed both

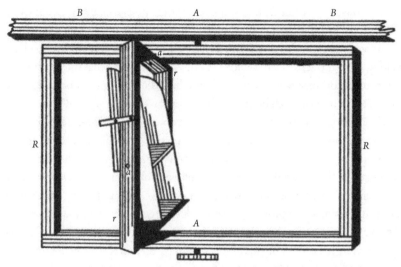

Figure 4.4 Rotational chair developed by Mach to test his theories on semicircular canal and otolith organ function. The chair could be centered over the vertical axis (A) so that just the semicircular canals were activated, or it could be moved off-center away from the vertical axis so that both the semicircular canals and the otolith organs were stimulated. In the off-center position, the subject could be turned in any direction or tilted about a horizontal axis (a). Source: From Mach E. *Grundlinien der Lehre von den Bewegungsempfindungen.* Leipzig: Engelmann, 1875.

linear and angular acceleration. Subjects perceived a turning sensation with the onset of acceleration, and this turning sensation persisted for 20–30 seconds after acceleration had ceased and a constant velocity rotation was achieved. The subject reported a sense of rotation in the reverse direction when the chair was decelerated and stopped, again lasting for 20–30 seconds after the stoppage.

Mach speculated that the angular acceleration was sensed by the semicircular canals, but unlike Breuer, he thought that it was not possible for the endolymph to actually flow within the canals because the tiny narrow canals would produce a very high degree of friction. (Remember that the entire inner ear is the size of the tip of one's little finger.) He suggested that the angular movement more likely would produce a pressure on the receptor organs in the ampulla of the semicircular canal. To convince himself of this, Mach performed experiments using closed glass pipettes of the size and form of the semicircular canal and a round channel in a brass plate covered with glass. He found that it was not possible for the fluid to move in these tiny circular tubes, so he concluded that the sensory receptor in the ampulla of the semicircular canal must have been stimulated by pressure because pressure stimulates the tactile nerves of skin. This issue as to whether or not there is actual endolymphatic fluid movement within the semicircular canal is still not completely resolved, although Breuer later came around to agreeing with Mach that there must be very little, if any, movement of the endolymph within these tiny canals. With his experimental rotational device for generating centrifugal force and with another device that he developed to produce pure linear acceleration along a linear track, Mach was able to convincingly show that there were separate receptors for sensing linear acceleration that, like Breuer, he concluded were located in two other small chambers in the inner ear—the utricle and the saccule.

Mach and Breuer were both aware of the problem that the linear acceleration sensors in the inner ear would have to differentiate between linear displacements of the head and changes in the direction of gravity that occurred with head tilt. Mach suggested the possibility of two different kinds of linear acceleration sensors, one for sensing linear head movements and one for sensing gravity, but Breuer believed that a single receptor could do the job. Breuer reasoned that all natural head movements are a combination of linear and angular accelerations, the former being sensed by the otolith organs and the latter by the semicircular canals so that simultaneous activation of the otolith organs and canals indicated to the brain that there was a combined linear and angular movement of the head (a natural head movement). On the other hand, static head position relative to gravity (head tilt) resulted only in activation of the linear acceleration sensors (the otolith organs). Of course, unusual situations such as traveling around a curve on a railroad or being spun on a centrifuge would confuse the brain and lead to an illusion of tilt (as occurred with Mach on his train ride and illustrated in Figure 4.3).

Breuer and Mach Work Together to Defend Their Theory

All in all, Breuer and Mach came to similar conclusions, with only small divergent details. They went on to become close friends, often working together to defend their theory, the Mach–Breuer theory, against doubters and detractors. Mach noted on several occasions that Breuer's animal experiments, which he was not able to carry out himself, provided the key support for their theory. It is interesting to consider how these two brilliant scientists with markedly different backgrounds came to similar conclusions about how the inner ear works at approximately the same time.

Breuer's medical training taught him a mechanistic view of science. He was convinced that every single anatomical detail has an important part to play in the overall function of an organ if only it is examined closely enough. His approach to understanding the function of the semicircular canals and otolith organs was to carefully study their structure, both at the gross and the microscopic level. He reviewed all of the prior knowledge on anatomy and physiology of the inner ear receptor organs and carefully dissected the inner ears of numerous animals to formulate his theory on how the inner ear works.

By contrast, Mach, with his background in psychophysics, developed his theory based on a perceptual observation—the fact that objects in the environment appeared tilted when going around a curve on a railroad track. Both investigators performed experiments on human subjects to test their theories, with Breuer relying on reflex eye movements (nystagmus) and Mach on the subjective report of motion perception. Their approaches complimented each other, making their theory more compelling.

Crum-Brown, the Model Maker

Remarkably, at approximately the same time, a third investigator working independently in Edinburgh, Scotland, came to the same conclusion regarding the function of the semicircular canals as Mach and Breuer. On January 19, 1874, Alexander Crum-Brown presented a preliminary communication to the Royal Society of Edinburgh describing his theory on how the semicircular canals of the inner ear work (Crum-Brown, 1874a). Although Crum-Brown had received an M.D. degree at Edinburgh University, he did not practice medicine but, rather, went on to study chemistry at London University, receiving his doctor of science degree in 1862. After a year of postdoctoral training in Germany, he returned to Edinburgh, where he was initially appointed as a lecturer in chemistry and then a professor in chemistry in 1869. Crum-Brown made numerous contributions to the field of chemistry; he is probably best known for his use of the symbol of two parallel lines to indicate a double bond. His breadth of knowledge extended well beyond science to include the study of philology, church history, and modern languages including Russian and Chinese.

Like Mach and Breuer, Crum-Brown surmised that movement of the fluid in the semicircular canals could explain the subjective sensation of rotation reported by subjects after starting and after stopping rotation. He developed a rotational devise similar to but less sophisticated than that of Mach to test his hypothesis on normal human subjects. He had blindfolded people sit on a stool mounted on a platform so that he could smoothly rotate each subject about the vertical axis and have the subject report on the sensation of rotation after accelerating to a constant velocity and then stopping. As with Mach, he noted that the sensation of rotation gradually subsided once the subject reached a constant velocity and then reversed direction and gradually subsided after the platform was stopped. He was also aware of the work of Goltz and Flourens, and he concluded that the semicircular canals in the inner ear were the likely organs for sensing angular rotation. Similar to Mach and Breuer, he speculated that rotation in the plane of a semicircular canal pair resulted in movement of the endolymph relative to the wall due to inertia "irritating" the nerve endings in the ampulla. The person's perception of rotation gradually decreased after a constant velocity was achieved or after stopping due to friction of the fluid against the membranous wall of the canal. Interestingly, he noted that the duration of this sense of rotation varied with different angles of head tilt that stimulated different combinations of canals. He attributed this difference in duration of sensation to differences in the diameter or degree of attachments of the membranous canals to the surrounding bone. We now know that this difference in the duration of sensation is due to differences in the brain processing of the signals coming from the horizontal and vertical canals and not due to the physical features of the canals.

Crum-Brown (1874b) developed an ingenious mechanical model to illustrate his theory (Figure 4.5). It consisted of two large wheels mounted side by side on a flat platform representing the semicircular canals on each side. Each wheel

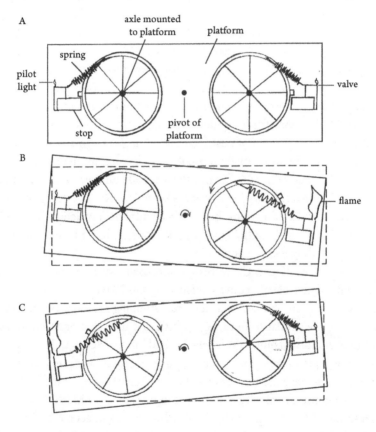

Figure 4.5 SCHEMATIC DRAWINGS MADE BY THE AUTHOR TO ILLUSTRATE THE KEY FEATURES OF CRUM-BROWN'S MODEL OF THE SEMICIRCULAR CANALS. In panel B, where the platform is accelerated in a clockwise direction about the central pivot, the wheel to the right moves counterclockwise due to its inertia stretching the spring and opening the valve so that the flame becomes bright. The wheel to the left cannot move because of the stop. In panel C, the platform accelerates in a counterclockwise direction and the wheel on the left moves in a clockwise direction, stretching the spring and opening the valve, producing a bright flame.

was limited to one revolution by a stop; rotation in the opposite direction was restricted by the stretching of a spring. An adjustable valve on each wheel opened as the springs stretched, and it closed as the springs relaxed. Gas was passed through pipes attached to the valves and ignited so that the brightness of the flame reflected the degree of stretching of the springs. Turning of the platform caused the wheels to turn in the opposite direction (due to their inertia), the springs to stretch or relax, and the valves to open or close. The changes in the intensity of the flames that resulted from stretching and relaxation of the springs represented the rate of firing of the nerves innervating the ampullae of the semicircular canals. When the flame was bright on one side, it was dim on the opposite side because the springs were attached to the wheels in opposite directions. Thus, he emphasized that the semicircular canals on each side sensed motion in opposite directions, allowing a blindfolded subject to distinguish between rotations to the left and to the right.

Crum-Brown had a lifelong interest in making models, having made a practical machine for weaving cloth before he had gone to school. A new contribution well illustrated by his mechanical model of the semicircular canals was the reciprocal functioning of the canals on the two sides. He concluded that the sensory receptor in the ampulla of the semicircular canal needed to sense movement of endolymph in only one direction because the paired semicircular canal on the opposite side sensed endolymph movement in the opposite direction. However, Breuer would later conclusively show that each ampulla sensed movement of endolymph in both directions. This explains why patients with only one inner ear can still sense rotations in both directions. Still, Crum-Brown's model provided valuable insight into how the paired semicircular canal system works. It anticipated the torsion-pendulum mathematical model of semicircular canal function developed many years later by Steinhausen (1931). Crum-Brown also noted that subjects usually were not bothered by rotation while blindfolded but often developed motion sickness when rotated in the light, particularly with the head tilted. He speculated that the conflicting sensory signals from the semicircular canals and visual system were the cause of the sickness. This so-called sensory conflict theory is still considered the best explanation for why people develop motion sickness.

Who Contributed Most to Our Current Understanding of the Vestibular System?

When the question is phrased in this manner, there is little doubt that Josef Breuer contributed much more to our current understanding of how the vestibular system works than Mach or Crum-Brown. Breuer's extensive writings on the anatomy and physiology of the vestibular receptors more than the 30 years after his initial presentation have withstood the test of time and, except for a few minor details, are still considered valid. For Mach and Crum-Brown, their work on the vestibular system was a brief interlude in careers focused on other areas. Crum-Brown mostly based his theory on published literature, and he personally performed only a few experiments to test the theory. He did not address the issue of linear acceleration sensors to compliment the angular acceleration receptors or how the sensory transduction in the inner ear might occur. With his model, he demonstrated the importance of the paired semicircular canals on the two sides, but he incorrectly concluded that each canal sensed motion in only one direction. Mach correctly surmised the presence of linear and angular acceleration sensors in the inner ear, but he focused only on the percept of movement and did not address the reflex eye movements (nystagmus) or the mechanism of sensory transduction. He believed that there were different "kinds of apparatus" for sensing head tilts and linear accelerations of the head. Like Crum-Brown, he concluded that each semicircular canal only sensed motion in one direction. Recall that Mach acknowledged that Breuer's animal experiments provided the critical support for the theory. Before we address Breuer's experimental work on the inner ear in detail in Chapter 6, we first address his background and training in Chapter 5.

References

Blackmore JT. *Ernst Mach: His work, life and influence.* Berkeley, CA: University of California Press, 1972.

Breuer J. Über die Bogengänge des Labyrinths. Vorläufige Mitteilung. *Anz Ges Ärzte* 1873;7:15–18.

Breuer J. Über die Function der Bogengänge des Ohrlabyrinthes. *Wien Med Jahrb* 1874;4:72–124.

Crum-Brown A. Preliminary note on the sense of rotation and the function of the semicircular canals of the inner ear. *Proc R Soc Edinburgh* 1874a;8:255–257.

Crum-Brown A. On the sense of rotation and the anatomy and physiology of the semicircular canals of the inner ear. *J Anat Physiol* 1874b;8;327–331.

Flourens P. *Recherches expérimentales sur les propriétés et les functions du système nerveux dans les animaux vertébrés.* Paris: Crevot, 1842.

Goltz F. Über die physiologische Bedeutung der Bogengänge des Ohrlabyrinthes. *Arch Physiol* 1870;3:172–192.

Grüsser O-J. J. E. Purkyne's contributions to the physiology of the visual, the vestibular and the oculomotor systems. *Hum Neurobiol* 1984;3:129–144.

Hoagland H. Quantitative analysis of responses from lateral line nerves of fishes, II. *J Gen Physiol* 1933;16:715–732.

Löwenstein O, Sand A. The activity of the horizontal semicircular canal of the dogfish *Scyllium canicula. J Exp Biol* 1936;13:416.

Mach E. Physikalische Versuche über den Gleichgewichtssinn des Menschen. *S Ber Akad Wiss Wien, math-naturw Kl* 1873;68(3):124–140.

Steinhausen W. Über den Nachweis der Bewegung der Cupula in der intakten Bogengangsampulle des Labyrinthes bei der natürlichen rotatorischen und calorischen Reizung. *Arch Physiol* 1931;228:322–328.

‖ 5 ‖

Breuer, the Renaissance Man

Upbringing and Formative Years

Breuer's father, Leopold, grew up in a poor devout Jewish family that lived near Pressburg, the ancient "coronation town" located between Budapest and Vienna (Hirschmüller, 1989). He attended a Jewish rabbinical school where the Talmud alone was taught. At age 15, Leopold fled to Prague, where he began the process of his self-education on "Western civilization." In 1836, four years before the birth of Josef, he was offered a position to teach religion in the Jewish community in Vienna, presumably through the mediation of his friend the Viennese rabbi Mannheimeer. During the following 22 years, Leopold showed himself to be a didactic, progressive Jewish scholar with an excellent all-around education. He maintained a running battle with the Orthodox Jewish community, which wanted its children's education to be limited to religious instruction and the learning of the Hebrew language, whereas Leopold felt strongly that no child should be deprived "of the benefits and demands of science and civic life." In 1840, when Leopold Breuer married Bertha Semler, he was 48 and she was 22 years old. Unlike Leopold, Bertha came from a well-established Viennese Jewish family, her father being a dealer of silk goods and her brother a wine merchant. Josef Breuer was born on January 15, 1842, in Vienna. He had hardly any recollection of his mother because she died soon after giving birth to her second child, Adolf, in 1844. Breuer noted, "Sometime later her mother [his grandmother], a brilliant and witty woman, came to live with us. She was to manage the household and act as a mother to the two motherless boys."

From all accounts, Josef Breuer had a happy, peaceful childhood. He did not attend primary school but was educated at home by his father, being able to read by age 4. In 1850, at age 8, Breuer entered the Akademisches Gymnasium, a secondary school in Vienna that placed particular emphasis on the natural sciences. Greek and Latin were standard courses, and in later years there was strong emphasis on philosophy with subjects such as analytical logic and empirical psychology. Josef Breuer passed the final examination from the Gymnasium in 1858 with distinction.

Although Josef Breuer had decided on a career in medicine while at the Gymnasium, he joined the Faculty of Philosophy, not the Faculty of Medicine, at the University of Vienna in 1858 because his father recommended that he take a year of general studies before entering medical school. Hirschmüller, Breuer's biographer, believed that Breuer's decision on a career in medicine was at least in part based on the fact that the best opportunities for a Jew in Vienna at that time were in the field of medicine. The chances for a Jew to secure an academic career were limited, and a career in public service was practically impossible. On the other hand, there were several Jews in high positions on the Faculty of Medicine in the university.

Austrian Jews could not vote or hold land prior to 1849, yet Jews dominated the intellectual life of 19th-century Austria. Being a Jew was a complex mixture of religion, race, education, and mores. The anti-Semitism that developed in the latter half of the 19th century was much broader and lacked the religious connotations of the earlier anti-Judaism. Although the noblemen and landed gentry who distained engaging in commerce themselves welcomed Jewish merchants and moneylenders, the Jews increasing wealth led to resentment and a scapegoat for gentile artisans, shopkeepers, and peasants who were sinking into poverty. Jewish families exhorted their children to study hard and excel at University at least in part to overcome prejudice. A good example was Freud's mother, Amalie, who was so anxious for her "golden Sigi" to succeed at school that she banned his sister from playing the piano in the evening so Freud could study in quiet (Johnston, 1972).

Breuer's Medical Training

Breuer began his medical training at the University of Vienna in the winter term of 1859–1860 (Figure 5.1). Despite the fact that the University of Vienna was considered to have one of the leading medical faculties in Europe, the physical structure was abominable. Lecture theaters were located all over the city, many of them being too small to hold all of the assigned students, and often students were required to walk long distances between lectures. The anatomy dissecting rooms were tiny, and students had to arrive hours in advance if they wanted a front seat at an anatomy lecture. Cadavers were in short supply, often being sold to the highest bidder. As many as 200 registered medical students would attend clinical lectures conducted at the bedside. Other than the required courses, the only elective course that Breuer signed up for was in the history of art. He chose not to enroll in an elective course in psychiatry.

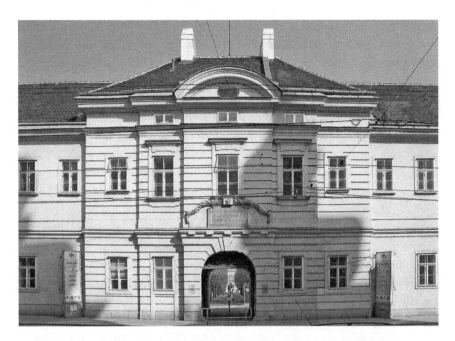

Figure 5.1 CONTEMPORARY IMAGE OF THE ENTRANCE TO THE VIENNA
GENERAL HOSPITAL (JOSEPHINUM) BUILT BY JOSEPH II IN 1784 AND MODELED
AFTER THE HÔTEL-DIEU DE PARIS. The Latin inscription above the entrance reads,
Saluti et Solatio aegrorum ("salvation and comfort of the sick"). Most of Josef Breuer's
medical lectures were in the Josephinum. Source: Photograph by Nicholas Wiest, Vienna
Austria, 2016.

Of the many fine members of the medical faculty, the three with the most
influence on Breuer were pathologist Carl von Rokitansky, physiologist Ernst
Brücke, and professor of clinical medicine Johann Oppolzer. Rokitansky was a
great believer in clinical–pathological correlation. He believed that an objective picture of disease emerged from thousands upon thousands of details
discovered on the dissecting table. Rokitansky taught that if the clinician
understood the pathological process, he could understand the clinical symptoms. Rokitansky was said to have performed more than 85,000 autopsies in
his career.

Ernst Brücke was credited with integrating German laboratory medicine with
Viennese bedside medicine. Along with Helmholz and Dubois-Reymond, he
founded the naturalism movement based on the hypothesis that an organism is
governed by no forces other than straightforward physical and chemical forces
as opposed to the prevailing vitalism movement, the notion of a supernatural
vital force driving all living beings. Brücke carried on a lifelong personal and
professional feud with the famous Viennese anatomist and vitalist, Joseph Hyrtl
(Wiest and Baloh, 2006).

In Oppolzer, Breuer found the ideal role model of a medical doctor. Oppolzer was known for his bedside manner that radiated confidence and optimism. He emphasized the healing powers associated with "the laying on of hands." Oppolzer was very supportive of his students and assistants, allowing them a large degree of freedom and encouraging their scientific work and training in the different subspecialties of internal medicine. After completing the minimal period of attendance required of a student, Breuer passed his examinations with distinction and was awarded the degree of Doctor of Medicine on July 1, 1864.

In February 1867, at age 25, Breuer obtained the coveted position of assistant physician to Oppolzer. Initially he received no payment as a second assistant but was entitled only to accommodation in the clinic. However, later that year, he became Oppolzer's first assistant with an annual salary of 420 gulden (approximately $210 at the time or $5,800 currently). Working in Oppolzer's clinic, Breuer was exposed to a wide patient population that included conditions under present-day subspecialties of neurology, otolaryngology, gynecology, and psychiatry. Breuer obtained an excellent broad medical training.

At that time, marriage was strictly prohibited for a young assistant physician. However, Breuer went ahead and married Mathilde Altmann, the youngest daughter of a Jewish wine merchant whose family belonged to the class of propertied Jewish trade people, on April 24, 1868. He entered a petition to the Ministry of Education on "acceptance of the marriage state" asking for an exception to the rule (Hirschmüller, 1989). The Ministry and the Professional College demanded that he promise to spend every other night in the clinic, but Breuer refused to give this assurance even though it meant the possibility of dismissal. In the end, a compromise position was accepted when he promised to live in the vicinity of the clinic.

Mathilde Breuer was a quiet, reserved woman who satisfied herself with raising her children and looking after her husband's social responsibilities. Their oldest son, Leopold Robert, was born in 1869. They went on to have four additional children, with the last one, Dora, being born in 1882. Robert took after his father and became a Doctor of Medicine, eventually becoming Chief Physician in the Hospital of the Jewish Community in Vienna, a position that he held until his death in 1936. Like Ménière's son Emile, Robert Breuer would go on to edit his father's letters.

Overall, Breuer's family life was a happy one, with the usual trials and tribulations of a man trying to balance his busy medical practice with the many responsibilities of a large family. In his autobiography, Breuer wrote (as quoted in Hirschmüller, 1989),

> When I can conclude this brief account of my life by saying that my
> home has always been a happy one, that my dear wife has given me 5

delightful and clever children, that none has been lost to me or caused me serious concern, then I may well claim to be a very fortunate man indeed. (p. 31)

He was indeed fortunate not to have lived to see two daughters die in the Holocaust: Dora took poison when she was about to be arrested by the Gestapo, and Margarethe died in a concentration camp.

Breuer Chooses Private Practice over Academic Medicine

In April 1871, Oppolzer died unexpectedly during a typhus epidemic, so Breuer lost his mentor and position. He was forced to leave the clinic and establish himself in the first district of Vienna as a general practitioner.

Why did Breuer end up in private practice rather than an academic position at the University? Before applying for an academic position, a young physician had to first submit his application for habilitation, which documented his training, academic distinctions, and evidence of scientific accomplishment. The habilitation document had to be reviewed by a professional college and by the Ministry of Education. During Breuer's assistantship with Oppolzer, he published only a few clinical papers in addition to his work on respiratory regulation with Hering that he performed in early 1868 in the Physiological Institute of the Imperial and Royal Josefs Academy. Although Breuer had the initial idea and approached Hering for his assistance and the use of his laboratory, Hering clearly had the major role in organizing and conducting their physiological experiments on the role of the vagus nerve in the reflex control of inspiration and expiration in animals (the Hering–Breuer reflex) (Ullmann, 1970). After his initial studies with Hering, Breuer did no further work in the field of respiratory physiology, probably at least in part due to the fact that Hering left Vienna for Prague in 1870. Breuer performed his work with Hering in early 1868, but he did not submit the work to the Academy until November of that year, probably because of the circumstances surrounding his marriage in April 1868. Presumably, Breuer did not consider the sum of his work to be adequate for habilitation at that time, and so he made no attempt at habilitation. When Oppolzer died in 1871, Breuer would likely have been appointed a locum tenens until a successor could be nominated if he had become habilitated.

After completing his innovative studies on the inner ear in 1873 and 1874, Breuer submitted his application for habilitation in December 1874. The number and quality of his publications were now more than adequate, and he was immediately accepted for the habilitation proceedings. He took his oral examination on February 6, 1875, passing with ease, and on February 13 he gave his test lecture on Basedow's disease (hyperthyroidism). The habilitation proceedings were considered complete on March 6, and the Ministry of Education confirmed habilitation in writing on March 20, 1875.

Breuer began his official career as a Privatdozent (licensed unsalaried lecturer) in the winter term of 1875–1876 with a course of lectures on diseases of the digestive organs presented on Saturday and Sunday from 11:00 a.m. to 12:00 noon. The timing of these lectures was dictated by his busy private practice. He went on to give a variety of different lectures during the next 10 years, at which time he suddenly resigned his lectureship in a letter to the Dean of the Faculty of Medicine in July 1885. This highly unusual move resulted from a complex series of events.

Breuer had a great deal of difficulty in obtaining appropriate patients for his lectures before the medical students (Hirschmüller, 1989). This was a common problem for lecturers in private practice because most of the appropriate patients for demonstration were in public hospitals. The rapidly increasing numbers of students and lecturers was limited by the scarcity of patients for clinical training. In order to obtain a professorship at the medical school, candidates (mostly lecturers) had to demonstrate adequate teaching credentials. One way for Breuer to overcome the problem in obtaining patients for his lectures would have been to apply for a post in a public hospital. However, these positions were rare and in great demand in Vienna. Another possibility would have been to accept a post in a provincial university and use that as a stepping stone to a post at Vienna University. Breuer was offered a professorship in internal medicine at Innsbruck, but he turned it down primarily due to the low salary. By this time, Breuer's private practice was flourishing and financial demands associated with his enlarging family were an important consideration. Breuer repeatedly applied for a Chief Physician position at different public hospitals in Vienna, and he even secured an additional title of Doctor of Surgery in 1877 because candidates for positions in the public service usually needed doctorates in both medicine and surgery. In April 1884, Sigmund Freud wrote to his wife Martha that "rumor has is that Breuer has again applied for the vacant position as Primarius [Chief Physician] in the hospital; I would be delighted if he succeeded, then I would do everything to become his Sekundararzt [assistant] and learn a lot. But he won't get it" (as quoted in Jones, 1961, p. 111). Why Freud was so sure that Breuer, despite his brilliant scientific productivity, would be turned down for the position is unclear, although it seems unlikely that it was entirely due to his lack of teaching experience. Any recommended appointments by the University had to pass through a series of government agencies. As Prospect Ménière found out, the process could be fraught with problems, particularly if the applicant had

had a negative interaction with any of the reviewers. Another issue that must be addressed is whether the growing anti-Semitic attitudes in the population as a whole could have been a factor in Breuer's repeated rejection for a University position. As Hirschmüller (1989) noted, "it is certainly true that in the mid-1880s being Jewish was not exactly a favorable incidental quality" (p. 28). The high rate of Jewish immigration from the east was raising concerns about "the Jewish problem" within the Viennese government. On the other hand, there were several non-Jewish members of the Medical Faculty, including the well-known surgeon Theodor Billroth, who strongly believed that Breuer should be offered a professorship. Billroth wanted to recommend Breuer for a professorship, but he was asked not to by Breuer himself because he apparently believed that it was a futile effort. Billroth is quoted as saying, "a Privatdozent [private lecturer] who never becomes an Extraordinarius [professor with tenure] bears a dagger in his heart until the day he dies" (Hirschmüller, 1989, p. 335).

Breuer made a clean cut with the university system by resigning his lectureship in 1885. Despite this, Breuer maintained close contacts with many members of the Medical Faculty at the University who became his friends and patients. Election to the Academy of Sciences in 1884, a rare accomplishment for a practicing physician, undoubtedly lessened the disappointment of not receiving a professorship at the medical school. Mach, Hering, and another longtime friend, Sigmund Exner, nominated Breuer for the Academy of Sciences.

Breuer, the Family Doctor

In many ways, Josef Breuer was the prototypical family doctor. His patients found him to be a caring friend as well as an outstanding diagnostician. Because of these qualities, his practice grew into one of the largest in Vienna. His list of patients and their families included some of the most prominent names in Viennese society (e.g., Ernst Fleischl von Marxow, Sigmund Exner, Sigmund Freud, and Johannes Brahms) (Hirschmüller, 1989). In addition to Billroth, he cared for a long list of eminent professors on the Faculty of Medicine, including Brücke, Cappozi, Frisch, and Schnabel. He was family physician to several of the "first Jewish families in Vienna," including the Wertheimstein and Gomperz families. These families were particularly known for their social gatherings of the intellectual elite of Vienna. Hirschmüeller commented that "there were hardly any Viennese scientists, writers, musicians, actors, painters or architects whom Breuer could not get to know at some time or other at these gatherings" (pp. 32–33) Breuer carried on a correspondence with one of his patients, Maria von Ebner-Eschenbach, for more than 27 years. Ebner-Eschenbach traced her ancestry to the Bohemian and Moravia aristocracy, although she was obviously in sympathy with the liberal thinking intellectuals of Breuer's social stratum. Not only was Breuer a medical advisor and personal friend to Ebner-Eschenbach but also his letters to her dealt with questions of science, literature, the history of art, philosophy, politics, as well as personal matters. Maria Ebner-Eschenbach wrote a short poem to Breuer expressing her feelings (as quoted in Hirschmüller, 1989):

> To Herr Doctor Josef Breuer
> my dear friend,
> the doctor to whom I commend
> my body, spirit and soul. (p. 34)

References

Hirschmüller A. *The Life and Work of Josef Breuer: Physiology and Psychoanalysis* [Transl of *Physiologie und Psychoanalyse in Leben und Werk Josef Breuers*, Verlag Hans Huber, Bern, 1978]. New York: New York University Press, 1989.

Johnston WM. *The Austrian Mind. An Intellectual and Social History 1848–1938.* Berkeley, CA: University of California Press, 1972.

Jones E. *The Life and Work of Sigmund Freud.* London: Basic Books, 1961.

Ullmann E. About Hering and Breuer. In: *Breathing: Hering–Breuer Centenary Symposium.* R Porter, ed. London: Churchill, 1970, pp 3–15.

Wiest G, Baloh RW. The personal and scientific feud between Ernst Brucke and Josef Hyrtl. *Otol Neurotol* 2006;27:570–575.

6

Breuer's Experiments on
the Semicircular Canals
and Otolith Organs

After his groundbreaking work in the mid-1760s, Breuer continued to perform experiments on the inner ear balance receptors in animals in addition to his busy medical practice and, at times, hectic family life. In part, he was driven by the need to respond to doubters of his theory on the function of the semicircular canals such as Benno Baginsky, who continued to claim that the semicircular canals had nothing to do with balance and that the findings of Flourens and Breuer resulted from injury to the brain rather than the inner ear (Baginsky, 1881). Breuer repeated his old experiments but refined the techniques to include the use of selective mechanical, thermal, and electrical stimulation of the crista of each semicircular canal. Breuer (1889) stated, "I believe that enough semicircular canals have been cut. . . . In the end we must use subtler methods than the ever popular cutting, splitting or burning of the canals for investigating the sensory organ which certainly exists in the vestibule" (p. 139). With regard to the otolith organs, the macules, Breuer had to perform pioneering experiments here because there was almost no literature on the subject at the time. As with the semicircular canals, he studied the macules of fish, reptiles, and birds and noted that all these creatures had three macules arranged in the planes of the semicircular canals, perpendicular to one another. By contrast, mammals had only two macules located in the utricle (horizontal plane) and saccule (vertical plane), again perpendicular to each other. He developed the concept of "slip" to describe the movement of the otoconial membrane over the underlying sensory epithelium that occurred with linear displacement or gravity (Breuer, 1891). Finally, he developed a mathematical model to hypothesize that in human beings there was only one combination of responses from the two macules on each side for a single head position in space.

Studies on the Semicircular Canals

Breuer carefully dissected the inner ears of hundreds of animals until he was able to conclude how the semicircular canals sensed angular movement and how they sent the signal on to the brain. When he was later criticized for the fact that he did not perform any experiments on mammals, Breuer stated (as quoted in Hirschmüller, 1989),

> So far as I am concerned, this omission is due to personal circumstances which I hope may be accepted as an excuse. I am a practicing physician. My time for experimentation is limited to the late evening and the night, and my laboratory is my home. I was able to experiment on pigeons, but radical operations involving mammals were out of the question. (p. 74)

Ironically, by concentrating his dissection on fish and birds, Breuer was probably better able to understand how the semicircular canals work than if he had focused on mammals. The large, highly developed semicircular canals of fish and birds were much easier to access and study than the tiny semicircular canals surrounded by dense bone found in most mammals.

As noted in Chapter 4, Breuer identified a gelatinous mass, the cupula, filling much of the semicircular canal ampulla (see Figure 4.1). In his subsequent studies, he observed that tiny hairs projected into the cupula from the cells at the base of the organ (hair cells) (Breuer 1897, 1903). With this new information, he modified his original hypothesis that the sensory cells were activated by bending of the hairs as endolymph moved over them to the idea that the endolymph movement resulted in a deflection or indentation of the cupula, which in turn resulted in bending of the hairs protruding into the cupula (Figure 6.1). He realized that the amount of endolymph flow must be tiny because deflection of the cupula is very slight. This slight deflection, however, would produce tension on the hairs on the side of the cupula toward the endolymph flow. Breuer recognized that the enlargement of the canal at the ampulla allowed this sensory structure to sense even very tiny currents of flow and also protected the delicate hairs from a sudden impact of endolymph movement.

Breuer performed a series of physiologic experiments on single ampullary nerves, clearly demonstrating that the induced nystagmus (head nystagmus in pigeons) was in the plane of the activated canal. He showed that the animal generated nystagmus in both directions when rotated in the plane of a single semicircular canal even after the opposite inner ear was destroyed. Breuer assumed that there were two types of receptors in each ampulla, one sensing movement of the hairs in one direction and the other sensing movement of the hairs in the opposite direction. The long-lasting after-sensation and nystagmus following

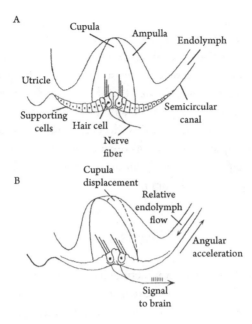

Figure 6.1 STRUCTURE AND FUNCTION OF THE CRISTA OF THE HORIZONTAL SEMICIRCULAR CANAL. In panel B, with angular acceleration in the plane of the canal, the endolymph moves in the opposite direction, displacing the cupula and bending the hairs protruding into it from the underlying hair cells. The nerve terminals at the base are activated and send the signal on to the brain. In the horizontal canals, the kinocilia (tallest cilia) are lined up on the utricular side, whereas in the vertical canals the kinocilia are on the canal side.

starting or stopping of angular rotation were explained by Breuer based on a continuing deflection of the cupula with a gradual return to its resting position (like a pendulum, as noted previously).

Recall that prior attempts to activate single semicircular canals had been crude, relying on cutting or burning the canal. Critics suggested that these crude stimuli were actually activating the brain, only millimeters away, defending the generally held view that head movements were sensed through a direct pressure effect on the brain. Breuer overcame these criticisms by using a magnifying glass to carefully activate a single ampullary nerve without any possibility of brain stimulation or injury (Breuer, 1903). In addition to electrical stimuli, Breuer used a cold probe to activate the ampullary nerve and induce nystagmus. He stated, "It still remains uncertain as to whether the effect is due to the cooling of the nerve endings or to endolymphatic flow" (Breuer, 1889, p. 139). He was clearly aware that thermal stimulation of the canal could produce powerful currents within it. As discussed in Chapter 9, Breuer's work with thermal stimuli on the dissected semicircular canal of the pigeon would be at the center of the controversy regarding Bárány's Nobel Prize for the discovery of the caloric reaction.

Breuer went on to conduct a series of experiments using cocaine to anesthetize the ampullary nerve from a single semicircular canal. Since the work of Flourens, there was debate regarding whether damage to a semicircular canal produced nystagmus (head or eye) by stimulation or by paralysis (loss) of function. Breuer convincingly showed that the nystagmus resulted from loss of function because it occurred after the ampullary nerve was anesthetized with cocaine. Furthermore, he showed that electrical stimulation did not result in nystagmus if the ampullary nerve was previously paralyzed with cocaine, thus conclusively proving that electrical stimulation had its effect on the ampullary nerve and not indirectly on the brain.

Ewald's Laws

At the same time Breuer was conducting his experiments on selective electrical stimulation of the ampullary nerve from the semicircular canals in pigeons, Ewald developed his ingenious method for inducing endolymph flow in a single semicircular canal of a pigeon (Ewald, 1892). Ernst Julius Ewald followed Goltz as professor of physiology in Strasbourg, Austria. He used his "pneumatic hammer" to systematically induce endolymph flow toward the ampulla (ampullopetal) and away from the ampulla (ampullofugal) (Figure 6.2). Ewald carefully dissected out each semicircular canal in the pigeon and made two tiny openings in the bony wall of the canal, leaving the membranous canal uninjured. In the hole furthest from the ampulla, he inserted a metal plug that pressed the membranous labyrinth against the opposite bony wall, effectively blocking the canal and preventing endolymphatic flow past that point. In the hole closest to the ampulla, he inserted a capillary tube with a tiny glass piston inside (his pneumatic hammer). The capillary tube was attached to a rubber hose and a rubber bulb. Squeezing the rubber bulb caused the piston to compress the membranous labyrinth, resulting in ampullopetal (toward the ampulla) flow, whereas relaxation of the bulb released the compression and caused ampullofugal (away from the ampulla) endolymphatic flow. He found that ampullopetal and ampullofugal endolymph flow in the same canal produced nystagmus in opposite directions consistent with Breuer's earlier findings. Ewald formulated two key observations that later became known as Ewald's first law and second law of semicircular canal function. Ewald's first law stated that the endolymph flow was in the direction of the slow phase of induced nystagmus. The second law stated that ampullopetal endolymph flow in the horizontal semicircular canal resulted in greater nystagmus response than ampullofugal endolymph flow, whereas in the anterior and posterior canals, ampullofugal endolymph flow resulted in greater nystagmus response than ampullopetal endolymph flow.

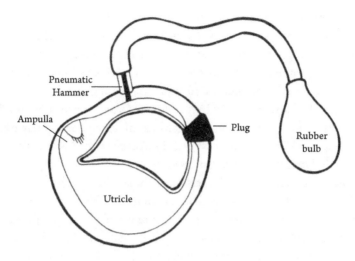

Figure 6.2 EWALD'S PNEUMATIC HAMMER. Ewald drilled two small openings in the bony wall of the semicircular canal careful not to injure the membranous canal. He placed a plug completely blocking the lumen of the canal in the opening farthest from the ampulla. He fitted a small cannula with a moveable plunger, "pneumatic hammer," into the second opening between the ampulla and the plug. A rubber bulb attached by a rubber hose drove the hammer forward and backward with compression and relaxation of the bulb. Compression of the bulb caused the endolymph to flow toward the ampulla (ampullopetal), and relaxation caused it to flow away from the ampulla (ampullofugal). Source: Ewald JR. *Physiologische Untersuchungen über den Nervus octavus.* Bergmann: Wiesbaden, Germany, 1892.

Although Breuer and Ewald were in complete agreement regarding Ewald's first law, Breuer suggested that Ewald's pneumatic hammer might have damaged the sensory receptors in the ampulla, tearing the delicate hair cells and thereby possibly producing the observed asymmetry in response. This controversy regarding Ewald's second law persisted for many years until it was shown to be essentially correct based on recording from the afferent nerves from the semicircular canals in several different animals. This asymmetry between the ampullary response to petal and fugal endolymph flow is the basis for a simple bedside clinical test (the head thrust test) to identify the loss of semicircular canal function on one side (Halmagyi and Curthoys, 1988).

The Breuer–Von Cyon Feud

Just as Ménière experienced when he suggested that vertigo could originate from the inner ear, there were vigorous attacks on the Breuer–Mach theory of semicircular canal function. The alternate leading theories on semicircular canal function were that either the semicircular canals played some part in perceiving the direction of sound (an acoustic function) or the semicircular canals were important for programming of motor movements in three-dimensional space. Although the proponents for an acoustic function for the semicircular canals held onto their views through the turn of the century, essentially denying all of the conclusive experiments by Breuer, Mach, Crum-Brown, and Ewald, their numbers were rapidly diminishing. Regarding this group, Breuer remarked in a letter to Mach in 1891, "There must be a limit, even to the thickness of thieves" (as quoted in Hirschmüller, 1989, p. 68).

The most vocal critic of the Breuer–Mach theory was the physiologist Eli von Cyon. Von Cyon's theory was essentially an extension of that initially proposed by Flourens. Von Cyon characterized the semicircular canals as "peripheral organs of spatial sense" with each pair of semicircular canals corresponding to a single dimension. In his extensive writings, von Cyon dismissed the Breuer–Mach theory as "a proliferation of weeds" (Hirschmüller, 1989, p. 70). Misunderstanding Breuer's observations, von Cyon claimed that he was the first to ascribe the function of spatial perception to the semicircular canals and that Breuer was negligent in not properly referencing him. Breuer vigorously disputed this claim, pointing out that his and Mach's initial work was conducted between 1873 and 1875, whereas von Cyon's first published work that characterized the semicircular canals as "peripheral organs of spatial sense" was published in 1877 (von Cyon, German translation in 1888). Furthermore, he criticized von Cyon's basic hypothesis that the semicircular canals provided a spatial sense because this was the function of the otolith organs and not the semicircular canals that were designed to sense angular rotation. He concluded that von Cyon's work consisted of one misunderstanding after another: "In circumstances like these, where the author gives an inaccurate account of another's position and then criticizes his misrepresentation there can be no point in detailed refutation of the criticism" (as quoted in Hirschmüller, 1989, p. 71). Apparently, von Cyon had some significant political clout because in a letter to Ernst Mach written in April 1908, Breuer mentioned that in 1897 he had difficulty getting a paper published in the *Archives of General Physiology* because the editor felt himself obliged to von Cyon in some way. Breuer summarized his feelings toward von Cyon with a quotation from Paul Heyse (as quoted in Hirschmüller, 1989):

> Ungrudging recognition is sweet,
> but it is a joy now and then
> to roundly call an impudent charlatan
> a rogue. (p. 71)

Clearly, Breuer did not suffer fools, and he was more than ready to defend himself whenever he believed that he was unjustly maligned.

Studies on the Otolith Organs

In 1873, after presenting his theory on the function of the otolith organs in the utricle and saccule in sensing linear displacement and head tilt, Breuer left these organs aside and focused on the semicircular canals for the next 10 years. A report by American physician William James, brother of the novelist Henry James, titled "The Sense of Dizziness in Deaf-Mutes" and published in the *American Journal of Otology* in 1882, rekindled Breuer's interest in the otolith organs. James noted that the majority of deaf-mute patients completely lost their sense of spatial orientation under water because they were deprived of all tactile and proprioceptive sensation. Drowning is a potential consequence, particularly if they dive into deep water. These findings conclusively supported Breuer and Mach's theory on the function of the otolith organs of the inner ear to sense the linear acceleration of gravity. Breuer began a series of detailed anatomical descriptions of the otolith organs of fish, frogs, birds, and some mammals because there was relatively little information in the literature about the structure of these organs (Breuer, 1891). He observed that, similar to the sensory receptor in the ampullae of the semicircular canals, the otolith organs had tiny hairs projecting up into the overlying otolithic membrane (Figure 6.3). He also observed that the otolith organs of the utricle and saccule were approximately perpendicular in mammals, with the utricular organ being approximately in the plane of the horizontal semicircular canal and the saccular organ midway between the planes of the posterior and anterior canals (in the sagittal plane). As he did with the semicircular canals, he used his detailed anatomical findings to deduce the function of these organs. As noted previously, he concluded that linear head displacements or head tilts (which changed the direction of the gravity vector) would cause the otolithic membrane to "slip," bending the hairs that were projecting into it and stimulating the underlying sensory receptor (Figure 6.3B). He speculated that the "direction of slip" due to head displacements or changes in the direction of gravity acting on the otolith organs takes place in one direction only. He believed that the structure of the otolith organ was ideally suited for his proposed function: bending of the underlying hairs in the direction of slip of the overlying membrane.

As discussed in Chapter 4, the apparent tilt of the perceived vertical under the influence of a centrifugal force (going around a curve in a train) suggested to Mach that there must be a sensory receptor for linear acceleration in the head (see Figure 4.3). Because Mach was primarily interested in psychophysics, he thought that this illusion was explained by the "sensibility of the body as a whole." Because of his interest in reflexive eye movements, however, Breuer wondered whether this illusion of tilt might be associated with a reflex rotation of the eyes. To prove this hypothesis, Breuer got together with Aloys Kreidl, a Czech-born physiologist

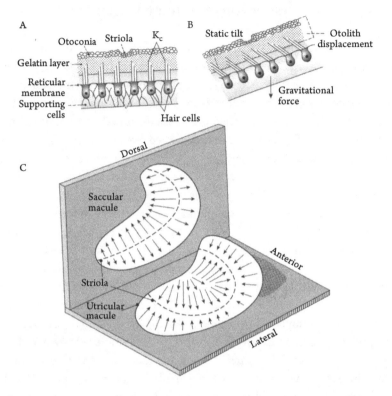

Figure 6.3 THE OTOLITH ORGANS (MACULES). (A) Structure. (B) With head tilt, the otolithic membrane is displaced due to the effect of gravity on the heavy otoconia. This causes the hairs to bend, activating the afferent nerve terminals just as in the case of the crista of the semicircular canals. (C) Orientation of the saccular and utricular macules. Arrows indicate the direction in which the kinocilia (K_c) point. Source: Adapted from Barber HO, Stockwell CW. *Manual of Electronystagmography.* CV Mosby, St. Louis, 1976.

working in Vienna, to perform a series of experiments on human subjects using Kreidl's rotatory chair that could be moved from the center of rotation, similar to that developed by Mach (Breuer and Kreidl, 1898) (see Figure 4.4). Kreidl, who is best known for his work showing that electrical stimulation of the hypothalamus activated the sympathetic nervous system, was one of the first to accept Breuer's theory on otolith organ function. In 1893, he conducted an ingenious experiment on crabs showing that displacement of the otolithic membrane resulted in compensatory postural changes (Kreidl, 1893). He placed iron filings on the otolithic membranes in crabs and then used a magnet to displace the otolithic membranes and produce the reflex postural movements.

A year earlier, he had used his rotational device to show that deaf-mute patients without functioning otolith organs did not experience an inclination of the subjective vertical axis—that is, an illusion of tilt—when they received centrifugal acceleration (Kreidl, 1892). Breuer and Kreidl (1898) used the same rotational device to measure eye rotations associated with the illusion of vertical tilt during centrifugal acceleration in normal subjects. To measure the eye rotation, they used an afterimage that was produced by means of a very bright vertical light (an incandescent wire) that was flashed onto the retina prior to rotation. Because this afterimage was transiently fixed to the retina, any rotation of the eye induced by the centrifugal acceleration would result in a tilt of the afterimage. They were able to measure the degree of tilt of the afterimage by having the subject cover the afterimage with a movable pointer.

The degree of eye rotation was then given by the angle between the pointer and the true vertical. As Breuer predicted, they were able to document rotation (torsion) of the eye when the subjects were rotated off-center with the head facing either forward or backward so that the resultant of the acceleration due to gravity and the centrifugal acceleration was in the frontal plane (as in Figure 4.3). Breuer and Kreidl used the analogy of an ice skater racing around a sharp corner who fully compensates for the centrifugal acceleration by leaning inward. They asked why wouldn't the eye muscles behave in a similar way? Both are reflex movements driven by the centrifugal acceleration on the otolith organs resulting in exquisitely timed motor responses proportional to the degree of centrifugal acceleration.

Overview of the Inner Ear Sensory Receptors

Overall, Breuer developed a simple basic concept to explain how the inner ear vestibular receptors work. All receptors responded to a shear force associated with acceleration, angular in the case of the semicircular canals and linear in the case of the macules (compare Figures 6.1 and 6.3). This shearing force results in a bending of the tiny hairs projecting into the cupula or the otolithic membrane, which in turn results in a change in the firing rate of the sensory nerves supplying these sensory organs. One organ responds to angular acceleration and the other to linear acceleration or gravity based on the surrounding structures. In the semicircular canals, the endolymph and cupula have a specific gravity of approximately 1 and therefore are not responsive to linear acceleration or gravity. Because of the shape of the canal, angular movement results in displacement of the endolymph–cupula system bending the hairs protruding from the underlying sensory membrane (see Figures 4.1 and 6.1). The otolithic membrane is a heavy structure due to calcium carbonate crystals (otoconia) imbedded in its surface so that it is sensitive to the direction of gravity or to applied linear accelerations, both of which bend the underlying hairs and generate a nerve signal proportional to the magnitude of the stimulus (see Figure 6.3). Although Breuer never used the term shear force, his so-called "shear theory" has proven to be correct in subsequent experiments in which nerve firing activity has been correlated with the direction and magnitude of applied force.

At this point, it is useful to consider some of these pioneering observations in light of our current knowledge. The hair cell is the key element in the inner ear that transduces the forces associated with head acceleration into nerve action potentials (Vollrath et al., 2007). A bundle of nonmobile cilia protrude from the cuticular plate at the apex of each hair cell (Figure 6.4). The height of the cilia increases stepwise from one side to the other, and next to the tallest cilia is the kinocilia. It protrudes from the cell cytoplasm through a segment of the cell apex lacking a cuticular plate. The tips of the cilia are connected by tip links attached to mechanosensory ion channels that open and close as the tip links stretch and relax (reminiscent of spring opening and closing the gas valve in Crum-Brown's model). Deflection of the cilia toward the kinocilium opens the mechanosensory channels at the tips, causing an influx of potassium and depolarization of the resting membrane potential. This opens voltage-gated calcium channels at the base and releases the excitatory neurotransmitter glutamate activating the nerve terminals at the base. Bending of the cilia in the opposite direction produces the reverse effect—closing of the channels and hyperpolarization of the hair cells. The stimulus for activating the hair cell cilia is a force acting parallel to the top of the cell resulting in a bending of the cilia (Breuer's shearing force). The stimulus is greatest when the force is directed along an axis that bisects the bundle of cilia and goes through the kinocilium (Figure 6.4, insert) (Hudspeth and Corey, 1977). As Breuer noted, a force applied to the cell surface (a compression force) would have no effect.

In the sensory epithelium of the semicircular canals, the cristae, all of the hair cells are lined up in the same direction—with the kinocilium on the utricular side in the horizontal semicircular canal (as in Figure 6.1) and on the canal side in the vertical canals. This explains Ewald's observation that endolymph flow toward the utricle (ampullopetal) in the horizontal semicircular canal leads to increased nerve firing, whereas it leads to decreased nerve firing in the vertical canals. Some of the mechanosensory channels are open when the cilia are in the straight up resting position, leading to a continuous baseline firing of the nerves. Bending of the cilia toward the kinocilium increases the baseline firing, and bending of the cilia away from the kinocilium decreases the baseline firing. The presence of baseline firing that is modulated by endolymph flow in opposite directions explains how a single semicircular canal can perceive angular rotation in both directions even when its partner on the other side is damaged (as Breuer observed). Because the resting firing rate can only go to zero with cilia deflection away from the kinocilium, whereas it can increase several-fold with

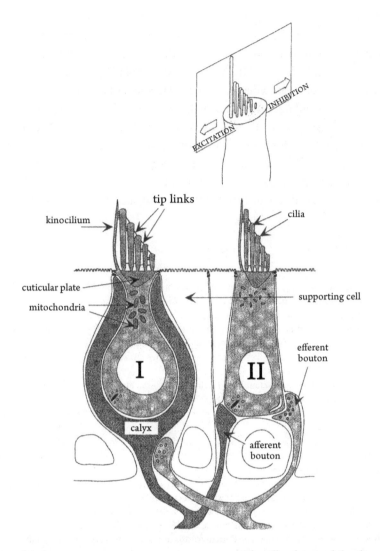

Figure 6.4 SCHEMATIC DRAWING OF HAIR CELLS. A bundle of nonmobile cilia protrudes from the apex in a staircase arrangement directed toward the longest kinocilium. Type I cells have an afferent nerve challis (calyx) surrounding the cell, whereas type II cells have afferent bouton nerve endings at the base. Both types receive efferent signals from the brain via bouton endings. Insert illustrates the relationship between the direction of force and maximum hair cell activation. Source: From Baloh RW, Honrubia V. *Clinical Neurophysiology of the Vestibular System*. 3rd ed. New York: Oxford University Press, 2001.

cilia deflection toward the kinocilium, there is a dynamic asymmetry in each hair cell's firing rate. This explains Ewalds observation that in the horizontal canal ampullopetal endolymph flow resulted in greater ampullary nerve firing than ampullofugal endolymph flow, whereas the reverse occurred in the vertical semicircular canals.

The situation is more complex in the otolith organs, where the sensory epithelium (the macule) is a curved structure bisected by the striola, a distinct curved zone running through the center dividing the macule into two parts. The hair cells on each side of the striola are oriented in opposite directions (the kinocilia are on opposite sides) so that displacement of the otolithic membrane either excites or inhibits the set of hair cells on each side of the striola (see Figure 6.3C). Groups of hair cells whose kinocilium is oriented with the same vector of excitability form functional units that cover all possible positions of the head in three-dimensional space. However, the majority of the units in the utricular macule are oriented in the horizontal plane, and the majority of those in the saccular macule are oriented in the vertical plane.

References

Baginsky B. Über die Folgen von Drucksteigerung in der Paukenhöhle und die Function der Bogengänge. *Arch Anat Physiol Abt* 1881:201–235.

Breuer J. Neue Versuche an den Ohrbogengängen. *Arch Physiol* 1889;48:139–152.

Breuer J. Über die Function der Otolithen-Apparate. *Arch Physiol* 1891;48:195–306.

Breuer J. Über Bogengänge und Raumsinn. *Arch Physol* 1897;68:596–648.

Breuer J. Studien über den Vestibularapparat. *S Ber Akad Wiss Wien math-naturw Kl* 1903;112:315–394.

Breuer J, Kreidl A. Über die scheinbare Drehung des Gesichtsfeldes während der Einwirkung einer Centrifugalkraft. *Arch Physiol* 1898;70:494–510.

Ewald JR. *Physiologische Untersuchungen über den Nervus octavus.* Bergmann: Wiesbaden, Germany, 1892.

Halmagyi CM, Curthoys IS. A clinical sign of canal paresis. *Arch Neurol* 1988;45:733–735.

Hirschmüller A. *The Life and Work of Josef Breuer: Physiology and Psychoanalysis* [Transl of *Physiologie und Psychoanalyse in Leben und Werk Josef Breuers,* Verlag Hans Huber, Bern, 1978]. New York: New York University Press, 1989.

Hudspeth AJ, Corey DP. Sensitivity, polarity, and conductance change in the response of vertebrate hair cells to controlled mechanical stimuli. *Proc Natl Acad Sci USA* 1977;74:2407.

James W. The sense of dizziness in deaf-mutes. *Am J Otol* 1882;4:239–254.

Kreidl A. Beitrag zur Physiologie des Ohrlabyrinths auf Grun von Versuchen an Taubstummen. *Arch Physiol* 1892;51:1119–1150.

Kreidl A. Weitere Beiträge zur Physiologie des Ohrlabyrinths. *S Ber Akad Wiss Wien math-naturw Kl* 1893;102:149–173.

Vollrath MA, Kwan KY, Corey DP. The micromachinery of mechanotransduction in hair cells. *Annu Rev Neurosci* 2007;30:339–365.

von Cyon E. Les organes périphériques du sens de l'espace. *Compt Rend Acad Sci Paris* 1877; 85:1284.

7

Breuer's Contributions to Psychiatry and Philosophy

Josef Breuer was a practicing physician who saw many patients with psychiatric symptoms. In that role, his job was to solve patient problems using whatever means at his disposal. He was a scientist and philosopher, but at his core he was a physician. His foray into the field of psychiatry can be directly traced to his patients, one in particular—a bright, young girl who became ill while she was nursing her sick father whom she adored.

Anna O, who is discussed in more detail later, exhibited a range of bizarre neurological symptoms that began with an intense cough followed by attacks of convergence spasm and double vision misdiagnosed as lateral rectus palsy. Breuer initially made a diagnosis of "tussis hysteria," classifying his patient as mentally deranged (Hirschmüller, 1989). At the time, doctors who cared for patients with hysteria in Vienna were called neuropathologists (not to be confused with current doctors who specialize in postmortem examination of the brain). A wide range of therapies were used, including special diets, "antihysteria drugs" (valerian and asafoetida), narcotics, hydrotherapy, and electrotherapy, none of which were very effective. Moritz Rosenthal and Moriz Benedikt were the leading neuropathologists in Vienna at the time. Rosenthal believed that hysteria resulted from an ill-defined structural abnormality of the spinal cord, whereas Benedikt considered it a functional abnormality—an impaired capacity for excitation within the nervous system.

Breuer made the chance observation that when his young patient was in a relaxed "autohypnotic state" she would relate the events that occurred at the time a particular symptom began, and remarkably after describing these events the symptom disappeared. Thus, Breuer arrived at a new treatment method, later called the cathartic method. The philosophical concept of catharsis, a purgation of emotions through art, can be traced back hundreds of years to Aristotle's principle of tragedy. With his extensive background in the classics, Breuer was well aware of Aristotle's work.

To understand how Breuer's chance observation led to the development of psychoanalysis, however, one must first understand the complex relationship that developed between Breuer and Sigmund Freud. Freud later wrote (Freud, 1925; English translation, 1963),

> Nothing in his education could lead one to expect that he [Breuer] would gain the first decisive insight into the age-old riddle of the hysterical neurosis and would make a contribution of imperishable value to our knowledge of the human mind. (p. 22)

Freud's Early Work in Neuroanatomy

Breuer first met Freud in approximately 1877 when both were working in the laboratory of Ernst von Brücke, the physiologist mentioned in Chapter 5 who greatly influenced Breuer's career (Wiest and Baloh, 2003). Freud had expressed a keen interest in the anatomy of the brain, particularly the brainstem, and Breuer encouraged Freud to perform a series of studies on the root fibers of the acoustic nerve. Freud used Weigert's staining technique, a standard method to stain the myelin sheaths on nerve fibers, to follow the central projections of the auditory nerve. In a series of three short publications, Freud erroneously concluded that the nucleus of Deiters was a third acoustic nucleus, despite prior studies showing that fibers to Deiters nucleus remained intact after sectioning the peripheral auditory nerve (Figure 7.1). We now know that Deiters nucleus is one of the main brainstem vestibular nuclei. Interestingly, Freud showed Breuer some of his anatomical preparations, but apparently Breuer did not suggest the possibility that Deiters nucleus was a vestibular nucleus even though he had previously mentioned the presence of vestibular nerve branches in the eighth cranial nerve in his famous 1874 paper, in which he first described how the semicircular canals work (see Chapter 4). In his autobiography, Freud (1925; English translation, 1963) described his relationship with Breuer at that time as follows: "He became my friend and helper in my difficult circumstances. We grew accustomed to share all our scientific interests with each other. In this relationship the gain was naturally mine" (p. 19).

Anna O. and the Beginnings of Psychoanalysis

The young girl with hysteria mentioned previously was the focus of Breuer and Freud's famous book, *Studies on Hysteria*, the starting point for the development of psychoanalysis (Breuer and Freud, 1895; English translation, 1955). She was given the pseudonym Anna O. in the book. Freud's biographer, Ernest Jones, revealed her real name, Bertha Pappenheim, in 1953, much to the consternation

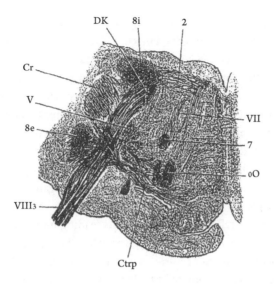

Figure 7.1 FREUD'S ILLUSTRATION SHOWING THE TRANSITION OF THE THIRD PORTION OF THE ACOUSTIC NERVE (VIII3) INTO THE FIBERS OF DEITERS NUCLEUS. Freud stained the medulla of fetuses with a method first introduced by Flechsig that depends on the fact that myelination of nerve fibers in different cerebral pathways reach maturity at different times. The method allows direct observation of the course and connections of nerve tracts that would be impossible to see in the mature brain. 8e, external acoustic nucleus; 8i, inner acoustic nucleus; DK, Deiters nucleus (Deiters kern); V, trigeminal nucleus and fibers; Cr, corpus restiforme; 2, fibers from 8i to the raphe; Ctrp, corpus trapezoides; 7, facial nucleus; VII, facial nerve; oO, superiorolive (obere Olive). Source: From Freud S. Ueber den Ursprung des N. acusticus. *Monatsschrift fuer Ohrenheilkunde* 1886;20:245–251, 277–282.

of her family and friends. Probably more has been written about Bertha than any other single patient in medical history. The obvious question is how could a family practitioner whose background was rooted in basic physiology and internal medicine become involved with such a patient. It is not entirely clear how Breuer became Bertha Pappenheim's doctor, although most likely he was already the family doctor for the Pappenheims, who were a prominent Jewish Viennese family. As noted previously, in 1880, while caring for her critically ill father, Bertha began developing a series of neuropsychiatric symptoms beginning with episodes of double vision followed by facial twitching and transient right arm anesthesia and paralysis. Other symptoms and signs rapidly followed, including severe occipital headaches and muscle spasms in all of her extremities. She had periods during which she would speak only in English or not speak at all. Breuer followed her carefully with daily visits, noting marked mood changes. The patient went into a serious crisis after her father died, and she became very dependent on Breuer's regular visits. On one occasion, Breuer found her in an "autohypnotic state" during which he was able to persuade her to recount events in her past history leading up to her illness. "Quite suddenly, she was awake, docile, cheerful, oblig-ing" Breuer observed (as quoted in Hirschmüller, 1989, pp. 86–87).

She improved so much that Breuer felt comfortable leaving her for his summer holidays. When he returned, he found her to be in a "wretched" state so that he again began an intensive daily therapy. He found that when the patient reported a specific circumstance when one of her many symptoms first occurred, her dis-cussion and description of the circumstance was followed by disappearance of the symptom. Using this basic strategy ("cathartic method"), Breuer systemati-cally achieved an abolition of most of her symptoms. However, the symptoms tended to return, and Breuer began to develop doubts regarding the success of his treatment strategy. He then began for the first time to use hypnosis in an attempt to get the patient to relive the psychic events leading up to her symptoms. He again noted a dramatic response, although as before, her symptoms continued to come and go with crisis after crisis. It is not entirely clear how Breuer developed his hypnotic technique, although he had seen Moriz Benedikt perform hypnosis in Oppolzer's clinic in 1868. However, at the time, he shared the prevailing skep-ticism, calling it "animal magnetism," and he questioned whether it should be used in a medical clinic (Hirschmüller, 1989). Later, he became more accepting of the concept as several close friends, including philosopher Franz Brentano, developed a keen interest in hypnosis. Charcot was already using hypnotism to treat hysteria in Paris in the 1870s. By 1880, Breuer had a broad understanding of hypnosis and was in position to tap into that knowledge when confronted with the unique circumstances of Bertha's treatment.

Bertha's treatment was obviously very draining, and Breuer began to have doubts about whether he was the appropriate person to continue her treat-ment. However, when he attempted to arrange for others to take over her care, she invariably went into a crisis. Finally, in the summer of 1882, Breuer con-vinced her mother that she should be admitted to the Bellevue Sanatorium at Kreuzlingen on Lake Constance. This marked the end of Breuer's formal treat-ment of Bertha, but he continued to maintain an interest in her case through contacts with the family. Despite the impression in *Studies on Hysteria* that Bertha was cured of her illness with Breuer's treatment, she continued to have relapses and was hospitalized on several occasions at the Vienna City Psychiatric Hospital between 1883 and 1887. Even later in life, she continued to have relaps-ing symptoms despite becoming a successful writer and working as a social worker (Hirschmüller, 1989).

Breuer and Freud and *Studies on Hysteria*

Breuer first told Freud about Bertha Pappenheim in November 1882, approxi-mately 5 months after he stopped treating her. It would be more than a decade, however, before they published her case history first in a preliminary communication in 1893 and in the book in 1895. As noted previously, Freud met Breuer in Brücke's laboratory, but at that time Freud had little interest in clinical medicine. After Freud joined the General Hospital as a young physician in 1882, Breuer became his clinical mentor and financial patron. Breuer was approximately 14 years older than Freud and probably saw himself as a father figure. In 1885, Freud received a travel scholarship and spent 6 months working with Charcot in Paris, where he observed Charcot treat numerous patients with hysteria. When Freud returned to Vienna, Breuer helped him set up a practice in "Neuropathology" at the University of Vienna. Over the following years leading up to the publication of *Studies on Hysteria*, Breuer worked with Freud on numerous patients, but he left the psychiatric aspects to Freud and concentrated on the medical aspects.

Why did it take so long for Breuer and Freud to publish Bertha's case history? The simple answer is that it took that long for Freud to convince Breuer to go ahead with the publication. Breuer had moved on. He had many other projects, including his vestibular work and his busy practice. He continued to see occasional psychiatric patients, but he referred them to Freud for their psychiatric care. There is no evidence that he ever used the cathartic treatment method again. Breuer did have concerns that it would be difficult to camouflage Bertha's identity in any publication, but most problematic to Breuer with regard to a joint publication was Freud's emphasis on sexuality in his theory on the cause of hysteria. Breuer was aware of and did not disagree with the widely held view that hysteria could result from frustrated sexual desires, but he was uncomfortable with making sexuality the center of their theory on cause. From Freud's point of view, he believed that Breuer's reluctance to publish was connected with the disturbing experience of a sexual attraction that developed between Bertha and Breuer during her treatment. In an attempt to alleviate Breuer's concerns, Freud told him about a woman patient who suddenly flung her arms around his neck during therapy, which he attributed to a transference phenomenon, "love transference," commonly associated with treatment of hysteria.

Freud biographer Ernest Jones went even further and suggested that Breuer had developed a countertransference for his patient and that Breuer's wife Mathilde suffered from it (Jones, 1961). He speculated that when Breuer became aware of his feelings for Bertha, he reacted with a mixture of love and guilt and broke off the treatment. Bertha reacted to the abandonment by developing a hysterical pregnancy that further horrified Breuer. Jones suggested that Breuer took his wife to Venice for a second honeymoon in an attempt to smooth over the problem. Hirschmüller, Breuer's biographer, could find no documentation of either the hysterical pregnancy or the trip to Venice, but he did believe that Bertha's treatment may have had an effect on Breuer's relationship with his wife (Hirschmüller, 1989).

The final version of *Studies on Hysteria*, published in 1895, consisted of four sections: (1) the mechanism of hysteria written by both authors; (2) five case histories—those of Bertha Pappenheim and four of Freud's patients; (3) a theoretical discussion by Breuer; and (4) a discussion of psychotherapy by Freud. The format was highly unusual considering that only the introduction was jointly written. One might wonder why they even bothered to publish jointly. No doubt Freud believed that publishing with Breuer was advantageous because Breuer discovered the method of treatment and his scientific reputation increased the likelihood of a good reception for the book (Hirschmüller, 1989). To get Breuer's cooperation, Freud agreed to keep the theme of sexuality in the background. Breuer, on the other hand, was loyal to Freud and wanted to support his work even though he had reservations. The central theme of Breuer's theoretical discussion in the book was "intracerebral tonic excitation" and the need for an organism to maintain constant intracerebral excitation. In a nutshell, he proposed that a "surplus of excitation" gained access to the sensory, vasomotor, and visceral apparatus, causing the observed pathological phenomena. The book received mixed reviews at the time, and Breuer's theoretical discussion was criticized for lack of specifics, particularly the lack of a mechanism to explain the excessive intracerebral excitation. Later, Freud speculated that the poor reception of Breuer's section of the book was the main reason Breuer ended their collaboration on hysteria.

The Friendship Between Breuer and Freud Dissolves

Breuer and Freud collaborated on numerous clinical cases and Breuer maintained an active interest in Freud's developing theories on psychoanalysis, but Breuer did not write any further on psychoanalysis. Breuer became increasingly uncomfortable with Freud's emphasis on the role of sexuality in the genesis of neurosis and his conclusion that hysteria resulted from "a sexual trauma of early childhood, which took the form of passive stimulation of the genitals" (as quoted in Hirschmüller, 1989, p. 169). Freud was obviously aware of Breuer's unease, but he continued to seek Breuer's opinion and he needed Breuer's acclamation. Breuer, by nature, was an empiricist who abhorred broad sweeping generalizations. He saw nothing as black and white but, rather, many different shades in between. By contrast, Freud was a zealot. With him, it was all or nothing. Criticism of any of his work was taken as criticism of his work as a whole. The final breakup occurred in the spring of 1896. In a letter to their mutual friend, Wilhelm Fleiess, Freud wrote, "I simply can't get on with Breuer at all; what I had to take in the way of bad treatment and weakness of judgment that is nonetheless ingenious during the past few months finally deadened me, internally to the loss" (as quoted in Hirschmüller, 1989, p. 188). For his part, Breuer felt betrayed by Freud but apparently tried to smooth over the dispute. Hirschmüller told of a story handed down by family members whereby in later years Breuer came across Freud on the street and went to greet him with open arms but Freud turned away and crossed to the other side of the street.

Breuer's Philosophical Beliefs

Breuer maintained a lifelong interest in philosophy, and he regularly corresponded with Theodor Gomperz and Franz Brentano, two of the leading philosophers of the time. In these letters, he discussed a wide range of topics, including vitalism, the existence of a soul, the theory of knowledge, Darwin's theory on the origin of species, and teleology as related to religion and science. Hirschmüller (1989) published what remained of these letters in an appendix to Breuer's biography.

A major issue facing the practicing physician in the late 19th century was how to reconcile the rapidly advancing scientific discoveries with the religious tradition of the medical profession. The earliest physicians were often priests who cared for the spiritual and physical needs of their patients. The ancient Greek physician Aesculapius founded a religious medical cult that flourished for more than 1000 years. Sick pilgrims flocked to the Grecian temples of Aesculapius, where they took part in a ritual called incubation. The god of medicine visited them during a dream state and would either heal them or prescribe specific types of treatment. Legend states that eventually the god of gods, Zeus, killed Aesculapius with a thunderbolt because he had revived the dead and thereby threatened the prerogatives of the deities. Throughout the Middle Ages, the close tie between religion and medicine was maintained in the medieval hospitals throughout Europe. The sick were cared for with the purpose of supplying their bodily wants and ministering to the spiritual needs until they were well enough to return to work. Because disease was considered to be due to evil humors brought on by past misdeeds, emphasis on the spiritual needs of the patient is easily understood. However, now that diseases could be explained by natural mechanisms such as bacteria, supernatural explanations were no longer required. On the other hand, despite the rapid advances that were occurring in science, science still could not explain most of the common disease processes. Being at the forefront of both the science and practice of medicine, Josef Breuer spent a great deal of time thinking and writing about the science/religion issue.

Breuer was foremost a scientist, and he was skeptical of traditional religious doctrine: "Those who do not possess science and art satisfy their need with religion, the doctrine of a God living outside the world, fashioned according to the image of men" (as quoted in Hirschmüller, 1989, p. 46). Many physicians find it difficult to maintain a cheerful disposition when dealing with the grim day-to-day details of the practice of medicine. Hirschmüeller wrote that "possibly the crucial factor in his personal philosophy of life is that, despite these experiences and his clear awareness of the dark side of existence, Breuer found reason to adopt an optimistic outlook" (p. 49). Breuer was well aware of the value of religion within society (as quoted in Hirschmüller, 1989):

> To those of us who are concerned particularly with the psychological aspect of religious phenomena and who have all but forgotten the "pious thrill deep down inside" of our childhood, religion does not mean something superhuman, something which is degraded and debased by human beings, but rather a product of the human spirit along with language and poetry, science and art. (pp. 47–48)

Although Breuer found it difficult to be satisfied with the beliefs of an organized religion, he did ruminate on the existence of God. His solution to the incompatibility of scientific and religious doctrine was to compartmentalize these two "products of the human spirit." He argued that the foundations for the evolution of the world are to be found in the structure of the "primeval cloud" that lies "beyond all possibility of experience" (Hirschmüller, 1989). Thus, science can explain the workings of the universe, whereas the primeval cloud was open to theological speculation for anyone so inclined. Breuer provided another analogy, recalling his difficulty understanding the mathematical concept of ∞ (infinity) as a child. He learned that ∞ could not be treated like other mathematical symbols but, rather, required its own separate rules. Breuer's religious beliefs were probably closest to Fechner's pantheism, the concept that God is the universe and all of its workings that Breuer called the religion of the 20th century. Breuer noted that Fechner presented his position "in such a way as to make it as credible as possible. This is certainly not a scientific approach, but it is the reason why he comes so close to my own position" (as quoted in Hirschmüller, 1989, p. 48).

Another closely allied issue facing the scientist and physician in the late 19th century was the mind/body issue. Psychology by tradition had been a branch of philosophy, a discipline separate from the physical world. However, with the growing realization that diseases of the mind are brain diseases, it became obvious that the brain was the anatomical seat of psychic function. There was a growing feeling among physiologists such as Brücke and Hering that physiologic methods would eventually solve the "mind problem" so that psychology would become obsolete. However, there were still strong proponents of the dualism theory that intellectual and material factors were functionally unrelated. Breuer believed that there were serious objections both to the monistic and the dualistic solutions but that monism was the better of the two solutions. Breuer's scientific training and clinical experience made it impossible for him to consider mind/body dualism because on a daily basis in his practice he saw how psychic events were dependent on the state of brain function. What irony that a scientist and physician with his background and beliefs would be considered a father of modem psychoanalysis.

As with every successful historical figure, Breuer possessed the personal qualities that assured his success. Hirschmüller (1989) noted that he was "a man of broad education who, on the basis of his intellectual capabilities, passed through the world with eyes wide open, bringing his finely discerning judgment to the important problems of his day" (p. 197). Breuer was not only well-read in the field of natural sciences but also had an extensive knowledge of the philosophical literature. Like Ménière, he had a particular interest in the classics, but he also read all of the modem writers, being particularly fond of Turgenev and H. G. Wells. His close friend, Hans-Horst Meyer, wrote (as quoted in Hirschmüller, 1989),

> Anyone who had the chance to talk with J. Breuer and to exchange ideas with him would not only be aware of the catholicity and depth of his reading in general; he would be amazed at the extent of Breuer's ability at any time to recall clearly and distinctly details which he once read or thought over. It made no difference whether the subject was historical and political events in whatever period or country, the teachings of the great thinkers and prophets or the works of poets and artists. (pp. 41–42)

Hirschmüller went on to write, "We might say that Breuer was a liberal in the best sense of the word, and that he experienced all the problems associated with the liberal outlook" (p. 197).

The Final Years

Breuer maintained an active interest in the function of the inner ear until the time of his death from prostate cancer on June 20, 1925. In his later years, he maintained a regular correspondence with the Dutch otologist, Adrian de Kleyn, who was performing a series of experiments on the role of the inner ear in the control of body posture and muscle tone. De Kleyn had trained with Rudolph Magnus, who conducted groundbreaking work on the role of the vestibular receptors on control of animal posture. An active topic in their discussion was the mechanism of stimulation of the hairs in the otolith organs, the macules. De Kleyn and several of his contemporaries thought that these organs were most likely activated by pressure as the heavy otolith membrane pressed down against the hairs. This was in contrast to Breuer's conclusion that the effective stimulus was a shear force bending the hairs in the "direction of slip" of the otolith membrane. In a letter to de Kleyn dated March 27, 1922, Breuer stated (as quoted in Hirschmüller, 1989),

> I realize clearly that I have generalized much too much from my findings with birds. The mammalian macula seems in fact to be almost flat; it does not have a cylindrical surface as is the case with birds. But I do not wish to concede my position as regards birds, for which the most sophisticated and accurate apparatus has been developed. (p. 272)

In a letter dated July 8, 1923, he suggested to de Kleyn that if he wished to contact him regarding the issues they had been discussing but in the meantime he (Breuer) had passed away, de Kleyn should pass his comments on to his son, Dr. Robert Breuer, who, although he was not an otologist, would certainly welcome such posthumous responses because of his interest in his father's affairs. He added, "I do not imagine that either event is imminent, the successful completion of inquiry or my death."

References

Breuer J, Freud S. *Studies on Hysteria*. Vienna: Deuticke, 1895. [Transl by J Strachey in collaboration with Anna Freud. New York: Hogarth, 1955.]

Freud S. *An Autobiographical Study*. Transl by James Strachey. London: The Hogarth Press 1959. (Original work published 1925)

Hirschmüller A. *The Life and Work of Josef Breuer: Physiology and Psychoanalysis* [Transl of *Physiologie und Psychoanalyse in Leben und Werk Josef Breuers*, Verlag Hans Huber, Bern, 1978]. New York: New York University Press, 1989.

Jones E. *The Life and Work of Sigmund Freud*. London: Basic Books, 1961.

von Ebner-Eschenbach M, Breuer J. *Ein Briefwechsel, 1889–1916*. Kann RA, ed. Vienna: Bergland Verlag, 1969.

Wiest G, Baloh RW. Sigmund Freud and the VIIIth cranial nerve. *Otol Neurotol* 2003;23:228–238.

ROBERT BÁRÁNY (1876–1936)

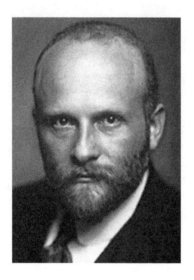

By the turn of the 20th century, as a result of the pioneering work of Ménière and Breuer, it was well known that vertigo and nystagmus could result from damage to the vestibular part of the inner ear. Despite his extensive studies of nystagmus in animals, however, Josef Breuer did not apply his findings to the clinical assessment of patients. It was Robert Bárány who recognized the value of nystagmus as a measure of vestibular function in patients. Bárány had a brilliant early career, working in the clinic of the pioneer otologist Adam Politzer at the University of Vienna, which culminated in his receiving the Nobel Prize for Medicine in 1914. However, in the aftermath of World War I and the controversy surrounding his selection for the Nobel Prize, Bárány left Vienna for Uppsala, Sweden, where he spent the last 20 years of his life in relative isolation.

8

Politzer's Otology Clinic and the Discovery of the Caloric Test

Adam Politzer graduated from the Vienna School of Medicine in 1859. As with his contemporary Josef Breuer, Politzer was influenced by the pathologist Rokitansky and the clinician Oppolzer (Majer and Kopec, 1985). After graduating from medical school, Politzer spent time in Paris working in the laboratories of Claude Bernard and Rudolf Konig, where he demonstrated oscillations of the auditory ossicles (tiny bones of the middle ear) after tonal stimulation (see Figure 1.1). He then went to London, where he had the opportunity to study the temporal bone collection of Joseph Toynbee. When he returned to Vienna in 1861, he became the first lecturer for otology at the University of Vienna through a unanimous vote of the College of Professors. It was not until 1873, however, that the administration decided to establish a stationary Clinic of Otology at the University of Vienna. There was a conflict because Josef Gruber had also set up a practice in otology at the University. In a typical bureaucratic decision, the administration decided to divide the directorship of the clinic between Gruber and Politzer (Majer and Kopec, 1985):

> In view of the fact that the Professors Dr. Gruber and Dr. Pollitzer [sic] have both been equally successful in the development of otology at the University of Vienna it is decreed that both be entrusted with the direction of the clinic in such a way that Prof. Dr. Gruber shall head the department for male ear patients while Prof. Dr. Pollitzer shall head the department for female ear patients. (p. 21)

The clinic was a single large ward partitioned in two, with Gruber's men's ward consisting of 11 beds and Politzer's women's ward consisting of 8 beds. In this single large room, operations were performed and large numbers of outpatients were examined and treated.

Politzer commented that "this division, which was unique in the history of medical departments, resulted in advantages which should not be underestimated. It was the trigger for a peaceful rivalry which was extraordinarily fruitful for science" (as quoted in Majer and Kopec, 1985, p. 17). Others did not consider the rivalry so peaceful. A young American physician, Alexander Randall, visited the clinic and noted that (as quoted in Stool and Sylvan, 1983)

> Politzer and Gruber, by the way, taught almost simultaneously in their wards—Politzer in the women's and Gruber in the men's, and each had one side of each adjoining room, so that when Politzer spoke rather contemptuously of a certain Josef Gruber and the latter in the like manner of Politzer, it was before a row of the other man's patients and with Wiethe often present as an assistant to each. Wiethe was supposed to be an oculist as well as an aurist and ought to have had a little dexterity, but he usually succeeded in making the nose bleed every time he did a Politzer inflation. (p. 347)

Politzer Maneuver

Politzer is probably best known for his discovery of a simple technique for inflation of the middle ear using an air bag (Politzer bag) (Figure 8.1). In describing his technique, Politzer noted (as quoted in Majer and Kopec, 1985),

> Condensed air can be blown through the Eustachian tube into the middle ear during an act of swallowing, the nasopharynx being closed on all side. The essential novelty of this method, by which it is distinguished from catheterization of the Eustachian tube, lies in the fact that the nozzle of the instrument to be used for condensation of air is introduced only into the anterior portion of the nasal cavity, and thereby the introduction of the catheter into the Eustachian tube, which is sometimes impractical and often disagreeable, is avoided. The most serviceable instrument for my method is a pyriform balloon, about the size of the doubled fist, which is furnished with a slightly curved tubular nozzle. The surgeon, standing on the patient's right, introduces the nozzle of the Politzer bag one centimeter into the corresponding orifice, and then compresses with the left thumb and forefinger the alae of the nose closely round the instrument. The patient is next told to perform an act of swallowing, and at the same moment the surgeon expels the air from the inflating bag with his right hand. By condensation of air, produced in the nasopharynx in this manner, the closure effected by the soft palate is forced open, and its vibrations give rise to a dull gurgling noise

which frequently, if not always, may be taken as an indication that the air has entered the middle ear. (p. 18)

This simple procedure could be performed by a general physician and even by the patient, providing the possibility to relieve the pain and discomfort associated with a variety of middle ear conditions. The procedure rapidly spread throughout the world.

The general accolades for Politzer's procedure further strained the "peaceful rivalry" within the Vienna Otology Clinic. Josef Gruber claimed that he, not Politzer, had originated the technique in 1862. In his *Textbook of Diseases of the Ear* published in 1870, Gruber referred to the "so-called" procedure of Politzer. Politzer in turn retorted with a caustic reply in his *Textbook of Otology* published in 1878:

> Since Jos. Gruber did not succeed—despite continual efforts—in denigrating the reputation which my process enjoys in Europe and America, he later (1870) undertook to suggest as a name for it "the passive valsalvan method" instead of "Politzer's method," which did not suit him. . . . Gruber's behavior appears all the more garish in that he did not shy from publicly declaring a modification of the closing of the pharynx in my method, which I adopted from Lucae, was a newly discovered method of his. (p. 174)

Politzer's textbook went on to become a standard work for the field for the next several decades. Five editions appeared up to 1908, and they were translated into French, English, and Spanish.

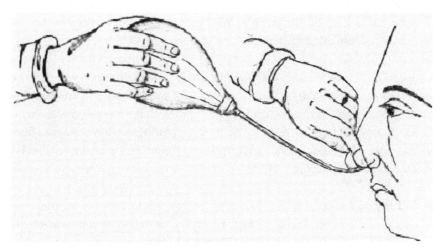

Figure 8.1 POLITZER'S MANEUVER (SEE TEXT FOR DETAILS). Original drawing from 1863.

Teaching in Politzer's Clinic

Above all, Politzer was noted for his teaching abilities, particularly his ability to inspire students with his untiring zeal for conscientious work. He was fluent in German, Hungarian, Bohemian, English, French, and Italian, so students from all over the world flocked to his clinic to study with the master. The American Randall (as quoted in Stool and Sylvan, 1983) described his experience at Politzer's clinic:

> With his mirror held by a handle between his teeth so as not to displace his scratch wig, he would spin around from one to another of his patients—"Have you zeen?" With crayon and stamp he would dash off a crude sketch of drum head (ear drum) details, fasten it to the patient's shoulder and make his demonstration of the conditions to be observed, broaden the illustration by reference to pictures on the wall or specimens in his cabinet and enlarge upon the meaning and treatment. (p. 347)

His surgical skills may not have been the greatest, but he did not lack in intensity. Randall described one of his operations as follows (as quoted in Stool and Sylvan, 1983):

> With little preparations and no anesthetic, he made his incision to the bone, fairly evacuating the pus, but opening a postauricular artery. Its spurt nearly washed him off his feet and utterly discombobulated him. Ligature and tenanculum were at hand, but hemostats were hardly yet known. He could not secure the spurter and would not let Woffler do so when he had summoned him from Bilroth's clinic. So you can imagine the feelings of our group as Woffler took the man by the ear and marched him off to the quiet of his own clinic. (p. 347)

Josef Gruber retired from the Otologic Clinic in 1898, the same year that two new rooms were added—a treatment room for outpatients and an operating room. Politzer retired from teaching in 1907, at which time he received from his students a valedictory address containing the signatures of 366 otologists from Europe, America, Asia, Africa, and Australia. In the address, it was noted that (as quoted in Majer and Kopec, 1985)

> nearly half a century has passed since you began lectures on otology; . . . those who received instruction and advice from you number in the thousands, how innumerable must be those who through your teachings have received their cure, health and indeed even life! (p. 31)

Robert Bárány Joins Politzer's Clinic

Robert Bárány began his training in Politzer's Otology Clinic in October 1903 after completing his surgical training at the Vienna General Hospital. During his general surgical training, Bárány became friends with Gustav Alexander, who already had been offered a position in Politzer's clinic. Alexander stimulated Bárány's interest in the vestibular apparatus of the inner ear and was influential in helping Bárány obtain his appointment in Politzer's clinic. These two young doctors spent long hours discussing interesting cases, reviewing the published literature on the vestibular apparatus, and planning future experiments.

A mundane job that both of them had to perform was to remove cerumen (wax) from the external ear canal of patients. The eardrum could not be visualized and hearing could not be tested if the ear canal was plugged with cerumen. It was well known in Politzer's clinic that one had to be extremely careful regarding the temperature of the water used to irrigate the ear canals in removing cerumen. When the canal was irrigated with cold water, the patient would experience vertigo with nystagmus, and occasionally there would be nausea and vomiting. The vertigo and nystagmus were minimal if the ear was irrigated with the patient sitting upright, whereas they were prominent if the ear was irrigated with the patient lying supine. The cause of this so-called "water-nystagmus" was unknown, but there was a general dictum that ears should be irrigated with water that was at or near body temperature.

Bárány Discovers the Caloric Test

Bárány later recalled (as quoted in Nobel Lectures, 1967),

> Among my patients [in Politzer's clinic] there were many who required syringing of the ears. A number of them complained afterwards of vertigo. Obviously I examined their eyes and I noticed in doing so that there was a nystagmus in a certain direction. I made a note of this. After a time, when I had collected about 20 of these observations, I compared them one with another and was amazed always to find the same note. I then realized that some general principle must be implied, but at the time I did not understand it. Chance came to my aid. One of my patients, whose ears I was syringing, said to me: "Doctor, I only get giddy when the water is not warm enough. When I do my own ears at home and use warm enough water, I never get giddy." I then called the nurse and asked her to get me warmer water for the syringe. She maintained that it was already warm enough. I replied that if the patient

found it too cold, we should conform to his wish. The next time, she brought me very hot water in the bowl. When I syringed the patient's ear he shouted; "But Doctor, this water is much too hot and now I am giddy again." I quickly observed his eyes and noticed that the nystagmus was in exactly the opposite direction from the previous one when cold water had been used.

. . . I remembered the water heater, and my astonishment, as a child, when I found the water just above the fire quite cold, but right at the top, the bath-oven was so hot it burned the fingers. The labyrinth (inner ear) now represented in my mind the water heater, a vessel filled with fluid. The temperature of this fluid is naturally 37°C—the body temperature. I squirt cold water at one side of the vessel. What must happen? What must naturally occur is that the water lying against this wall is cooled down; in this way it acquires a higher specific gravity than the surrounding water and sinks to the bottom of the vessel. On the other hand, water still at body temperature takes its place. If I syringe the ear with hot water, then the motion must be precisely contrary. But the motion of the fluid must be altered if I alter the position of the vessel. And it must be changed to the exact opposite if I turn the vessel through 180°. The test that had to be the crucial experiment for this theory occurred to me at once. If syringing the ear, be it with cold fluid or hot, succeeded in evoking nystagmus precisely opposite in direction for two positions of the head differing by 180°, then the theory must be the right one. (pp. 506–509)

Bárány knew that the bony wall of the horizontal semicircular canal was physically closest to the external ear canal and that temperature changes within the external canal would result in a change in the temperature chiefly in the short segment of the canal just behind the ampulla (Figure 8.2). The horizontal semicircular canal is approximately in the vertical plane when the subject is lying supine and the temperature change in the wall on one side of the canal would result in a change in the specific gravity of the endolymph within the canal. The cold water irrigation would make the endolymph slightly heavier, whereas a warm water irrigation would make it slightly lighter. Due to gravity, the endolymph would begin to circulate, away from the ampulla with cold water in the external canal and toward the ampulla with warm water in the external canal. When the subject is turned upside down (from supine to prone), the position of the horizontal canal with regard to gravity is reversed and so the effect of cold and warm water would be reversed (Figure 8.2, bottom compared to top). Subjects have minimal or no response when in the sitting position because the horizontal semicircular canal is in approximately the horizontal plane perpendicular to the gravity vector.

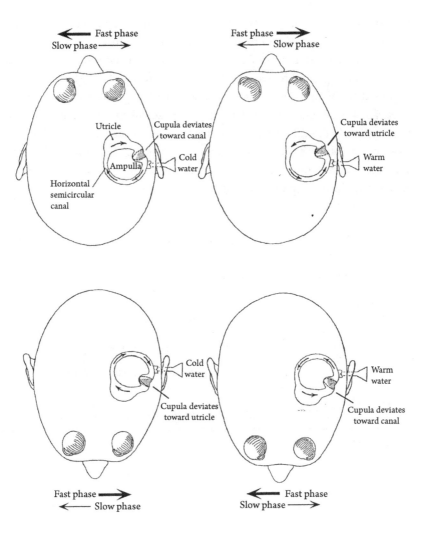

Figure 8.2 MECHANISM OF THE CALORIC RESPONSE. With the subject lying supine (top), cold water causes the cupula to deviate away from the utricle while warm water causes the cupula to deviate toward the utricle. If the subject turns upside down assuming the prone position (bottom), the direction of cupula deviation reverses, and the direction of the slow and fast components of nystagmus reverses.

Being a clinician, Bárány was immediately aware of the potential usefulness of the water nystagmus (caloric test) as a clinical test. It allowed a selective stimulation of each horizontal semicircular canal in sequence. As Breuer had previously noted, physiological rotational stimulation activated both horizontal semicircular canals simultaneously and patients with only one functioning canal still had nystagmus responses in both directions. Bárány now had a way to identify a malfunctioning canal on one side only (by comparing the duration of nystagmus after each caloric stimulus). He published the complete details of his caloric test first in a journal in 1906 and then in his book on the physiology and pathology of the vestibular system in 1907. Bárány's findings were considered to be pivotal in clinical otology, and he received international recognition. However, his colleagues at the Vienna University Clinic were less magnanimous in their praise of Bárány's accomplishments. Unlike the "peaceful rivalry" that had existed between Gruber and Politzer, the rivalry between Bárány and the other young assistants in Politzer's clinic was anything but peaceful. The details of the conflict in Politzer's clinic are addressed in Chapter 9 after a brief review of Bárány's formative years leading up to the conflict.

References

Bárány R. Untersuchungen über den vom Vestibularapparat des Ohres reflektorisch ausgelösten rhythmischen Nystagmus und seine Begleitererscheinungen. *Monatschr Ohrenheilk* 1906;40:193–297.

Bárány R. *Physiologie und Pathologie des Bogengangapparates beim Menschen.* Vienna: Deuticke, 1907.

Majer EH, S Kopec M. *History of Oto-rhino-laryngology in Austria: An Illustrated Document.* Vienna: Verlag Christian Brandstätter, 1985.

Nobel Lectures Including Presentation of Speeches and Laureates' Biographies. Physiology or Medicine. 1901–1921. Published for the Nobel Foundation in 1967 by Elsevier, New York, pp. 500–511.

Politzer A. *Lehrbuch der Ohrenheilkunde für practische Ärzte und Studierende.* Stuttgart: Enke, 1878.

Stool SE, Sylvan E. A historical vignette: Memoirs of an otologist's European study in 1883. *Am J Otol* 1983;4:346–349.

9

Bárány's Formative Years and the Conflict in Politzer's Clinic

Robert Bárány was born in Vienna on April 22, 1876, the first of six children to Ignaz and Maria Bárány. Both parents were of Jewish descent. Ignaz Bárány, who was born in Palota, Hungary, came to Vienna at age 14 after both of his parents died. He gave up his Hungarian citizenship and became an Austrian citizen in 1877, the year after the birth of his first son Robert. Ignaz Bárány worked as a manager in the lumber department of the Union Bank in Vienna for many years before becoming an independent lumber salesman. His wife Maria came from a prominent Jewish family in Prague. She was the fourth child of the well-known scholar Simon Hock, who had written extensively on the history of Judaism in Prague. Hock spoke and read 11 languages. Maria Bárány was clearly the dominant influence on young Robert Bárány. Bárány wrote (as quoted in Joas, 1997), "My mother was a tender mother and wife and a very clever woman. The talent for languages, love of truth and sharp critique are carried over from her father" (p. 20).

Robert Bárány was a bright student who consistently got high marks. Even as a child, he was quiet and aloof; he later wrote (as quoted in Joas, 1997), "I was often told when I was 14 and 15 years old that I was very self centered" (p. 20). As a child, Bárány contracted the most feared infectious disease of the time, tuberculosis. He was fortunate to recover, but the infection involved the bones in his leg and left him with an ankylosed knee joint. Bárány graduated from high school with honors in 1894 and decided on a career in medicine. According to Bárány (as quoted in Joas, 1997), "Studying medicine was the wish of my mother, who considered a physician a helper in spiritual and physical needs. I had no objections to this occupational choice, but also no great expectations regarding my future" (p. 21). Robert was the oldest of six siblings and the only one to receive a higher education. Of his three younger brothers, two became salesmen and the third a banker. One sister was a housewife, and the other died in childhood.

Bárány's Medical Training

Bárány began his medical training at the University of Vienna at the age of 18 in 1894. Unlike Ménière and Breuer, he did not receive a broad education in literature and the arts. Bárány wrote (as quoted in Joas, 1997),

> Until my twenty-first year, I considered myself totally without new ideas and not capable of independent new thinking. I did read some scientific literature and also criticized it. But it appeared to me, that I was capable only to critique the thoughts of others. (p. 22)

At age 21, Bárány had a revelation after reading a book by Arthur Schopenhauer: He was suddenly flooded with new ideas and new thoughts. He wrote (as quoted in Joas, 1997),

> I wrote down only such ideas and thoughts I never read or heard about before. An immense feeling of happiness flowed through me the entire day, and my confidence grew in an enormous way. I recognized that I am capable of performing productive work, to pursue new ways, independent of others, and I concluded I would devote myself from now on to scientific research. (p. 22)

From that day on, Bárány had a single-minded purpose in making new scientific discoveries. He became a prodigious worker who had few interests outside of his medical studies.

When Bárány graduated from the University of Vienna Medical School on April 2, 1900, medicine already had a strong scientific foundation and expectations for the new century were limitless. It was traditional at the time for new medical graduates to seek training abroad, so Bárány spent 2 years in German clinics studying internal medicine, neurology, and psychiatry. He studied psychology with Kraepelin in Heidelberg and with Pfi in Freiberg. While in medical school, Bárány attended lectures by Sigmund Freud and approached Freud about training with him, but Freud turned him down. Years later after learning that Bárány had received the Nobel Prize, Freud wrote (as quoted in Jones, 1961),

> The granting of the Nobel Prize to Bárány, whom I refused to take as a pupil some years ago because he seemed to be too abnormal, has aroused sad thoughts about how helpless an individual is about gaining the respect of the crowd. (p. 347)

What Freud meant by "too abnormal" is not entirely clear, but presumably he was referring to Bárány's aloof personality. Freud never received the Nobel Prize, but one of the first things that Bárány did after receiving his Nobel Prize was to use his prerogative as a Prize winner to nominate Freud for the Prize. When Freud received word of Bárány's nomination, he sarcastically noted to a friend that his chances of receiving the Nobel Prize increased from 6% to 7%.

After his experiences in Germany, Bárány decided that a career in neuropsychiatry was not for him (as quoted in Joas, 1997):

> Although I had the opportunity to become proficient in this field, I realized that this was not what I was seeking and when my application for recognition of my Austrian doctor's degree in Germany was rejected, I returned to Vienna with the intention of joining one of the so-called specialty areas. (p. 24)

He began his training with a general surgical residency at the Vienna General Hospital in the spring of 1902.

Source of Conflict in Politzer's Clinic

As mentioned in Chapter 8, during his surgical training, Bárány became friends with a young physician, Gustav Alexander, and it was Alexander who stimulated Bárány's interest in the vestibular system and helped Bárány obtain a position in Politzer's clinic. The two young assistants conducted several joint experiments on the vestibular system. However, when Bárány published his short book on the physiology and pathology of the vestibular system in 1907, he did not mention his collaboration with Alexander and did not cite any of Alexander's work (Figure 9.1). After rapidly putting the book together in a few weeks apparently because of concerns that others might beat him to the punch, Bárány had Politzer write the introduction but he did not show it to Alexander until he had sent it off to the publisher.

Alexander reacted angrily, claiming that Bárány left out many important references in his book and had failed to give credit to Alexander for his contributions to the overall work. In particular, he cited their collaboration on measuring eye rotations associated with head tilt and the fact that Bárány failed to quote a paper that they jointly authored (Alexander, 1907a):

> The author was not entitled to neglect my papers, which offered him a lot of encouragement and represent the basis for his further investigations at the Viennese Otology Clinic. If it was the intention of the author to make an original and independent impression, I have to enter my protest against this procedure. (p. 22)

Bárány responded point by point to Alexander's accusations. He admitted that he was wrong in not quoting the paper on ocular counter rolling by Alexander and himself but stated that the material described in his book was

A

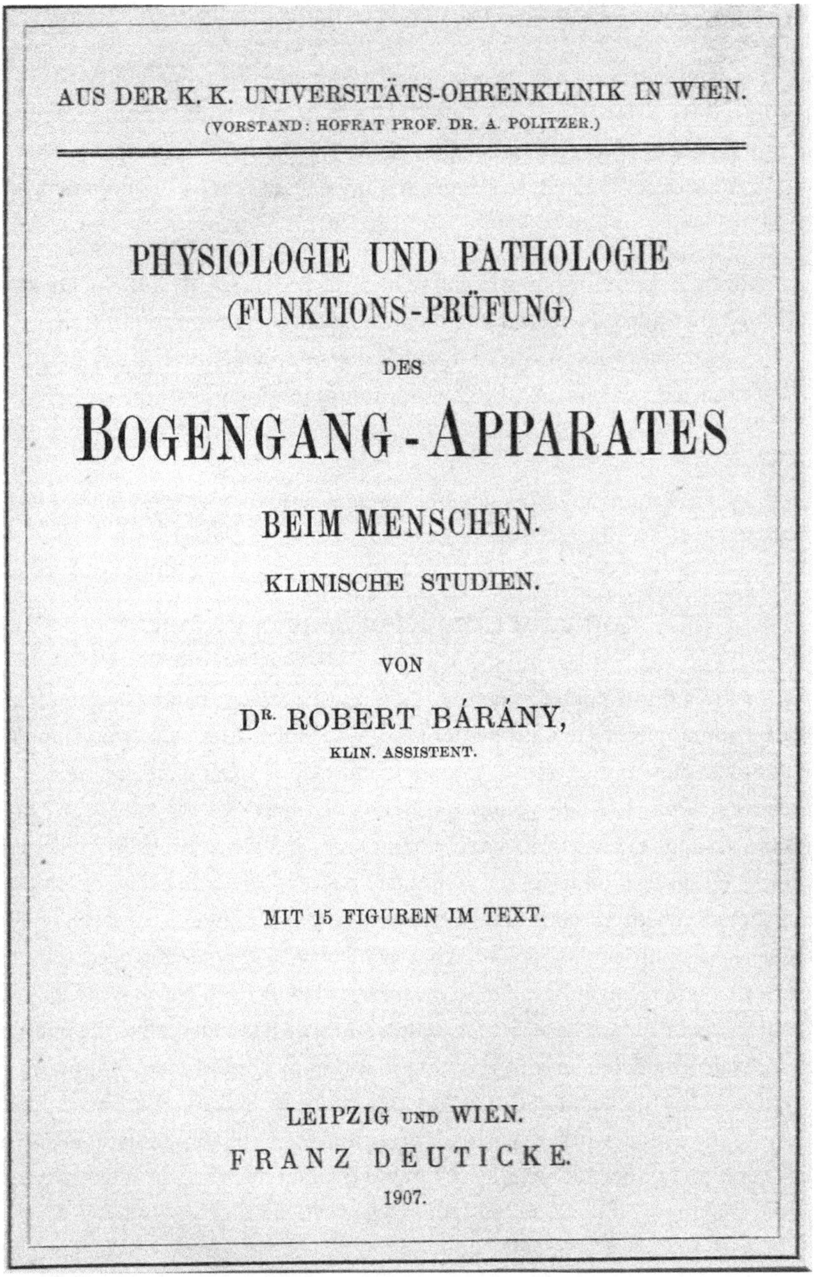

AUS DER K. K. UNIVERSITÄTS-OHRENKLINIK IN WIEN.
(VORSTAND: HOFRAT PROF. DR. A. POLITZER.)

PHYSIOLOGIE UND PATHOLOGIE
(FUNKTIONS-PRÜFUNG)

DES

BOGENGANG - APPARATES

BEIM MENSCHEN.

KLINISCHE STUDIEN.

VON

DR. ROBERT BÁRÁNY,
KLIN. ASSISTENT.

MIT 15 FIGUREN IM TEXT.

LEIPZIG und WIEN.
FRANZ DEUTICKE.
1907.

Figure 9.1 COVER (A) AND FIGURE 1 (B) OF BÁRÁNY'S FAMOUS 1907 BOOK ON THE PHYSIOLOGY AND PATHOLOGY OF THE VESTIBULAR SYSTEM. In panel B, Bárány demonstrates a method for identifying the planes of the three semicircular canals (SSCs) by placing the fingers of the left hand across the palm of the right hand. The fingers of the left hand represent the plane of the right anterior canal, the palm of the left hand represents the plane of the right posterior canal, and the palm of the right hand represents the plane of the right horizontal canal. a, ampulla of the horizontal SSC; b, ampulla of the anterior SSC; c, utricle; d, common crus of the anterior and posterior SSC; e, horizontal SSC; f, anterior SSC; g, posterior SSC. Source: From Bárány R. *Physiologie und Pathologie des Bogengangapparates beim Menschen*. Vienna: Deuticke, 1907.

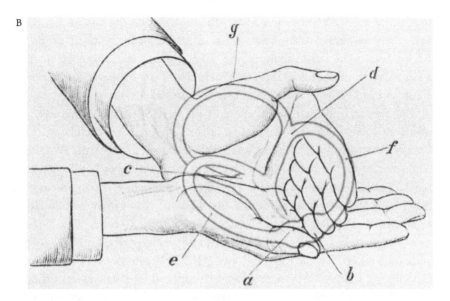

Figure 9.1 CONTINUED.

his own work independent of what he had done with Alexander (Joas, 1997). Alexander was not impressed with Bárány's explanation. "Long-winded explanations do not change injustice into justice," retorted Alexander (1907b, p. 23).

At approximately the same time, Bárány came into conflict with another young assistant in Politzer's clinic, Heinrich Neumann (Joas, 1997). Neumann claimed that he had suggested the critical cold and warm water experiments that led Bárány to discover the mechanism of the caloric response. During an ear operation that Neumann was performing along with Bárány and several other assistants, Neumann noted that the patient developed nystagmus when he began cleaning the horizontal semicircular canal with ether. According to those present, Neumann suggested that it would be interesting to perform experiments in healthy subjects and patients with defective inner ears using cold and warm water to stimulate the canal. Later when Bárány published the results of his experiments, Neumann was surprised that he was not informed of the experiments and not mentioned in the publication. When confronted with Neumann's accusations, Bárány claimed that he had already made the key discoveries regarding the caloric response before that operation took place.

Accusations Against Bárány

Malicious gossip began to circulate within the Otology Clinic and the University Hospital suggesting that Bárány's ideas were not original and that he had plagiarized others in his writings (Baloh, 2002). Bárány's aloof personality and his propensity for generating enemies with his caustic comments no doubt contributed to his problems. Although anti-Semitism was again on the rise in Austria, it is unlikely that anti-Semitism was a significant factor in the hostility toward Bárány because he was an agnostic who did not believe in Zionism. He married a Christian woman, and all three of his children were baptized. Furthermore, Neumann and Politzer were both of Jewish ancestry.

The rumors and innuendoes came to the surface when Bárány was proposed for Professor Extraordinum (professor with tenure) at the University of Vienna (Diamant, 1984). The honorary title was denied him by the Professor's Collegium of the Vienna Medical Faculty. The dean, Professor Tandler, gave the official indictment against Bárány. The heart of the matter was the accusation that Bárány did not discover the caloric reaction but, rather, this credit should go to Julius Eduard Hitzig and Josef Breuer. Hitzig was the German physician who discovered galvanic nystagmus when he passed an electrical current between electrodes placed on each mastoid area. He had previously shown in animal experiments that eye movements could be induced by stimulation of the ear with cold water, but this had already been known to occur in humans and it did not provide an explanation for the mechanism of the caloric response. Breuer had stimulated single ampullary nerves with a cold probe and suggested that the mechanism of stimulation could be either endolymph flow or direct activation of the ampullary nerve, but he claimed no priority for the "caloric reaction." Breuer found the matter distasteful and in a letter to the Dean of the Faculty of Medicine, he wrote, "I would not stoop to being instrumental in these proceedings even if my intellectual reputation had been harmed in any way as a result of Bárány's action" (as quoted in Hirschmüller, 1989, p. 76). He sent a copy of the letter to Bárány and gave him permission to publish it if desired. The Academic Senate, however, acknowledged Breuer's "excessive modesty" but continued with its proceedings against Bárány.

References

Alexander G. Physiologie und Pathologie des Bogengangapparates beim Menschen. Österreichische Ärzte-Zeitung 1907a;372:22–23.

Alexander G. Nachtrag zu meinem Referat über das Buch des Herrn Bárány. Österreichische Ärzte-Zeitung 1907b;398:23.

Baloh RW. Robert Barany and the controversy surrounding his discovery of the caloric reaction. Neurology 2002;58:1094–1099.

Bárány R. Physiologie und Pathologie des Bogengangapparates beim Menschen. Vienna: Deuticke, 1907.

Diamant H. The Nobel Prize to Robert Barany—A controversial decision? Acta Otolaryngol (Stockh) 1984;Suppl 406:1–4.

Hirschmüller A. The Life and Work of Josef Breuer: Physiology and Psychoanalysis [Transl of Physiologie und Psychoanalyse in Leben und Werk Josef Breuers, Verlag Hans Huber, Bern, 1978]. New York: New York University Press, 1989.

Joas G. Robert Bárány (1876–1936) Leben und Werk. Frankfurt am Main: Lang, 1997.

Jones E. The Life and Work of Sigmund Freud. London: Basic Books, 1961.

The War Years and Bárány's Decision to Leave Vienna

As the conflict in Politzer's clinic heated up and with the approach of World War I, Bárány volunteered for service in the army medical corps in keeping with his pacifist ideas. Although he could have been excused from military service because of his ankylosed knee, Bárány was swept up in the wave of patriotism prevalent in Vienna. He was immediately assigned as an army surgeon to a hospital in the fortress of Przemysl near the Russian border. The confident Austrians saw the war as their chance to revive the once proud Austro-Hungarian Empire. Unfortunately, their leaders were not up to the task. According to Winston Churchill, the octogenarian Emperor Franz Josef "had never declared a foreign war he did not lose, nor bent himself to a domestic policy which was not evidently failing" (Churchill, 1931, p. 7). The Austrian military fortunes were in the hands of Field Marshal Konrad von Hotzendorf, who was best known for his stern personality and the cruel treatment of his soldiers. Although Konrad and his Austro-Hungarian troops had some early successes after the outbreak of the war, the Third Austrian Army was soundly defeated by the Russian army at Lemburg, leading to a wild retreat back across the Russian plains with the Russian Cossacks in hot pursuit. Of the 900,000 Austrian troops in the battle, approximately 250,000 were killed or wounded and another 100,000 were taken prisoner. The fort at Przemysl where Bárány was stationed was right in the path of the chaotic retreat. A large number of the wounded soldiers were left at the fort, and the fort was reinforced with an army corps but the main army continued to retreat, leaving the fort at Przemysl in the middle of enemy territory.

The large influx of wounded soldiers provided Bárány the opportunity to work on his surgical skills. He performed up to 100 operations a day with a makeshift staff that included an anesthetist who formerly served as a swimming pool superintendent and masseur (P Bárány, 2013). He became particularly proficient in treating bullet wounds to the brain (Figure 10.1). At that time, it was customary to leave the wound open after the foreign body was removed. Bárány,

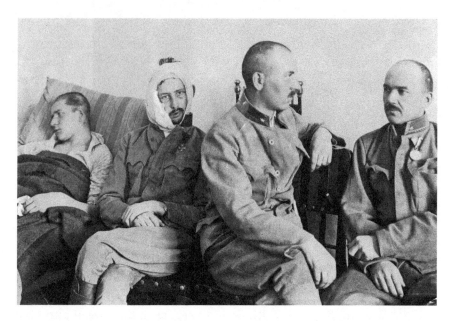

Figure 10.1 PHOTOGRAPH OF PATIENTS AT THE FORTRESS HOSPITAL IN PRZEMYSL. Source: Courtesy of Peter Bárány, MD, Stockholm, Sweden, grandson of Robert Bárány.

however, noted that he obtained better results if he cut away all damaged tissue, removed the bullet, disinfected the wound, and then closed the wound immediately (Bárány, 1915).

Przemysl had only approximately a 3-month food supply, and so it was just a matter of time before the Austrian garrison in the fort would have to capitulate. There was a successful effort to replenish the fort in October 1914, but subsequent efforts were repulsed and starvation forced the surrender of the huge fort in April 1915. Bárány was transported along with more than 100,000 other prisoners in cattle cars across the Russian steppe to Turkistan. Later, Bárány and the American neurosurgeon Harvey Cushing exchanged letters regarding their publications on treating head wounds during the war. Bárány gave a detailed description of his time in Russia in a letter to Cushing in April 1920 (as quoted in Carey, 2013):

> I came to the so-called worst location in Turkistan—Merv. The first impression is not enthusiastic for a Central European. Merv is an oasis in a sandy desert. The desert sand fills the streets and behind every vehicle dust rises as high as a house. I reported to the commander and was led to a villa already occupied by imprisoned doctors. We were 3 in a small room. No beds existed but I got one anyhow; no armoires. Obviously no table cloths, napkins, etc. I slept the first night in this room but it was so unbearably hot and the bedbugs bit me that I said to

myself, "I'll never do that again." Next evening I had my blanket spread out on the terrace of the villa's garden. I was warned about scorpions and indeed while my servant brought a glass of water he stepped next to my bed on something which proved to be a scorpion. I was very pleased because the others had heard about scorpions but had never seen one, now I was convinced that this would be the first and last I would ever meet. What was bothering me far more were mosquitoes which swarmed around me the first nights. Therefore when my bed arrived which had been cleared of thousands of bedbugs by setting fire to some petrol which had been sprinkled over the bed, I had a cage built over the bed with nets spread over it. That's how I slept in the garden for eight months. I still caught malaria but I've been clear of it for 3 years as it was only the simple tertian kind. All of my companions who were bitten untold many times caught the serious tropical malaria. (pp. 909–910)

Despite the difficulties that Bárány encountered as a prisoner of war in Turkistan, he expected and received special treatment consistent with his aristocratic background and medical prowess. His servant stayed with him throughout his travels. In Merv, Bárány was placed in charge of otolaryngology not only for all of the Austrian prisoners but also for the local Russians. Among his grateful Russian patients was the local mayor, who regularly invited Bárány to join him and his family for dinner (as quoted in Carey, 2013):

The Russian head physician said immediately that he knew my name from the medical literature since he was a self-taught ear specialist and he asked me if I would like to teach him and other doctors of the hospital about ear illness! That's how I could immediately continue my Viennese teaching in Turkistan! I received a special pavilion for my ambulance. All existing special instruments were given to me—regrettably there were only a few of them. I had, however, quite a bit to do. When it became slowly known that there was an ear specialist in Merv and particularly after I received the Nobel Prize some months later people came from far away to Merv. There are approximately half a million Russians in Turkistan and no ear specialist! (p. 910)

Bárány Receives the 1914 Nobel Prize in Medicine

It was during his stay in Merv that Bárány received the exciting news from the Swedish minister in St. Petersburg that he had been awarded the 1914 Nobel

Prize in Medicine for his work on the caloric reaction. Bárány responded with a telegram that read,

> Professor Gunnar Holmgren, Stockholm, Sweden, Have just been notified by the Swedish envoy about being awarded the Nobel Prize, which is highly gratifying for me. I am sending you—and please also forward it to the medical faculty of Stockholm—my most cordial thanks. Dr. Barany, prisoner of war. (Courtesy Gerald Wiest, MD, Vienna, Austria)

Bárány was initially led to believe that through the intervention of Prince Carl of Sweden, the Russians agreed to his release, but when he was moved to Taschkent, the officer in charge stated that he knew nothing about Bárány's release and that he would have to care for several officers and their wives before being sent to Kazan in central Russia. Bárány later found out that a Russian Red Cross delegate had agreed to Prince Carl's request for his release even though the delegate had no power to grant the release (as quoted in Carey, 2013):

> After a trip of one week I reached Kazan. The trip again was very comfortable. I sat in a second class wagon with my servant, and had a Russian soldier to watch over me but he acted like a second servant towards me and my luggage. At that time a trip of 8 days cost 50 rubles! I paid nothing but was informed about the cost by my fellow traveler. I arrived at Kazan Christmas Eve 1915 at 50 degrees of coldness. . . . Thanks to a Russian patient who had paid me with a fur coat I was quite well equipped. In Kazan I resided in a hotel but worked at the university. . . . After 5 months at Kazan I succeeded because of a stiff knee as a veteran to be sent home. My so often lamented knee became my savior because how it would have continued in Russia is hard to tell. Eight Austrian doctors who were still in Kazan during the revolution were shot by Czechoslovakian nationals. (p. 910)

Bárány obviously had mixed feelings regarding his memories of the war and his Russian imprisonment when he later wrote (as quoted in Nylen, 1965),

> In Russia, at least at that time, people's word of honor was regarded as nothing. I will, however, not express an unjust or hard opinion about the Russians in general. They have the weakness often not to stick to the truth, but even among them it is true, as my report shows, that I have met many kind-hearted and noble thinking human beings, as you can find among all peoples and races. (p. 317)

Remarkably, after traveling to Sweden and receiving the Nobel Prize, Bárány decided to invest nearly the entire amount of the prize in Austrian war bonds despite the fact that he was advised in Stockholm to leave the proceeds in a Stockholm bank. The bonds soon became worthless. Bárány 's close friend, Lorente de Nó, years later admonished Bárány "but, Professor, that was a senseless thing to do!" Bárány replied, "Well, I was an Austrian citizen and my country dearly needed all the help I could give" (personal communication, Lorente de Nó, 1975). His country and the University of Vienna in particular did not show the same loyalty to Bárány when he returned to the otologic department from Stockholm in 1916. There was open hostility from his colleagues within the otological department, and complaints were addressed to the Senate of the University of Vienna claiming lack of honesty in Bárány's writings.

Formal Charges Against Bárány

The circumstances were becoming intolerable in Vienna, and so when Bárány was offered the possibility to develop a new otolaryngological clinic in Uppsala, Sweden, in 1917, he immediately accepted the position. Prior to his departure, Bárány requested that the Academic Senate at the University of Vienna initiate a formal disciplinary proceeding regarding the accusations against him. The Academic Senate made its formal report in July 1918. The accusations consisted of four main points (Akten des Unterrichtsministerium, 1916/1917). The first point was the priority issue regarding the caloric test mentioned previously. The second accused Bárány of omitting the fact that he got the idea for the change in nystagmus direction with cold and warm water from Heinrich Neumann. The third point addressed the fact that he did not give proper credit to earlier investigators in his writings. Finally, the fourth point indicated that Bárány gave a false case presentation in Vienna in which he described a patient with a tumor in the cerebellar vermis (midline) but did not mention that there was also a tumor in the cerebellar hemisphere. Although this was bought to his attention after the Vienna meeting, he repeated the same case history at a lecture in London.

Regarding the first point, the Senate concluded that Hitzig was the discoverer of caloric nystagmus (1874) and that Breuer found the basic features of the response. Bárány's contribution was merely to describe the change of direction of nystagmus after application of cold and warm water that provided a physical explanation for the phenomenon. Regarding the second point, witnesses at the operation confirmed that Neumann suggested to Bárány the experiments with cold and warm water in normal subjects and patients. Regarding the third point, a witness described findings that Bárány claimed to have discovered but were already described by Mach and Breuer. Finally, witnesses confirmed that Bárány did not mention the cerebellar hemispheric tumor in either the Vienna or London lectures. The Academic Senate concluded (Akten des Unterrichtsministerium, 1916/1917),

> Dr. Bárány did not act scientifically correct, which was his duty as a faculty member, scientist and writer. His behavior demonstrates eminent carelessness in terms of the intellectual property of others. His failure cannot be attributed to a lack of skill or training, in contrast it is evident that Dr. Bárány represents a person of outstanding capabilities, diligence and training. The errors, failures and one-sided descriptions in his papers and lectures can only be explained by his addiction to enlarge his own merit at the expense of others. (p. 509)

Nobel Committee Response

It was not until 1920, however, that this formal list of accusations was submitted to the Medical Faculty of the Karolinska Institute in Stockholm, Sweden. The accusations were distressing to the Nobel Prize Committee, and they were carefully examined with the assistance of Professors H. Giertz and G. Holmgren. After extensive deliberations, the Nobel Prize Committee came to a completely opposite conclusion regarding the four points in the formal accusations (Diamant, 1984). The Committee concluded that Hitzig's and Breuer's work was purely experimental and that Bárány should be given priority for discovery of the caloric reaction. Regarding Neumann's suggestion to Bárány during an operation to test the effect of cold and warm water on the caloric reaction, the Committee discovered that Bárány had reported his findings regarding the change in direction of the caloric reaction several months earlier in a paper presented at an Academy meeting. The Committee concluded that Bárány had referenced other scientists working in the field in his many papers, and it could find no factual basis that Bárány deliberately ignored one of the brain tumors in the case that he had used to illustrate a point in several lectures.

Questions Regarding Bárány's Caloric Theory

Bárány's theory on caloric nystagmus came under fire from a different direction when a German otologist Kobrak (1918) found that irrigation of the ear canal with a small amount of water that was only one degree above or below body temperature was sufficient to produce a caloric nystagmus. Kobrak and others questioned whether such a small amount of heat could produce a significant change in the temperature of the horizontal semicircular canal and suggested that Bárány's caloric theory needed to be revised. However, at approximately the same time, G. F. Dohlman, who was working in Bárány's laboratory in Uppsala, designed a thermocouple that allowed direct measurement of the changes in temperature of the wall of the horizontal canal and showed that Kobrak's minimal irrigation did indeed produce measurable changes in temperature (Dohlman, 1935). The most severe crisis for Bárány's theory on caloric nystagmus would come years later when caloric responses to both cool and warm water were induced in normal human subjects in space (Clarke, Teiwes, and Scherer, 1993). Because there is minimal gravity in space, there must be some other driving mechanism for the caloric response. Some suggested that Bárány's Nobel Prize should be revoked (Stahle, 1987). As Breuer had previously surmised, however, the caloric response on earth is probably due to a combination of the specific gravity changes of the endolymph (Bárány's theory) and direct heating and cooling of the ampullary nerve. In space, the specific gravity effect is lost, but the effect from heating and cooling the ampullary nerve remains. This direct heating and cooling effect on the ampullary nerve accounts for only a portion of the caloric response on earth, however.

References

Akten des Unterrichtsministerium Über Robert Bárány. Österreich. Staatsarchiv., Doz. Dr. Collinger, *Abschrift* S.Z.509 ex 1916/1917.

Bárány R. Die offen und geschlossen Behandlung der Schussverietzungen des Gehirns. *Beitr Z Klein Chir* 1915;97:397–417.

Bárány P. Bárány and traumatic brain injury: Letter to the editor. *J Neurosurg* 2013;118:908.

Carey M. Response to letter to the editor by Peter Barany. *J Neurosurg* 2013;118:908–912.

Churchill WS. *The Unknown War.* New York: Charles Scribner's Sons, 1931.

Clarke AH, Teiwes W, Scherer H. Vestibulo-ocular testing during the course of a space flight mission. *Clin Invest* 1993;71:740–748.

Diamant H. The Nobel Prize award to Robert Bárány—A controversial decision? *Acta Otolaryngol (Stockh)* 1984;Suppl 406:1–4.

Dohlman G. Some practical and theoretical points in labyrinthology. *Proc R Soc Med* 1935;50:779–790.

Kobrak F. Berträge zum experimentellen Nystagmus. *Beitr Anat & c, Ohr* 1918;10:214.

Nylen CO. Robert Barany. *Arch Otolaryngol* 1965;82:316–319.

Stahle J. Robert Bárány—Ingenious scientist and farseeing physician. In *The Vestibular System: Neurophysiologic and Clinical Research.* Graham MD, Kemink JI eds. New York: Raven Press, 1987.

Bárány's Test Battery and the First Description of Benign Paroxysmal Positional Vertigo

In addition to his caloric test, Bárány developed an extensive battery of clinical tests of the vestibular system, most of which he outlined in his 1907 book on the physiology and pathology of the vestibular system. The basic concepts of his examination were to use the oculomotor responses (nystagmus) and postural responses (balance and past-pointing) to determine the functional status of the inner ear. He routinely performed a caloric test and a rotational test on all of his patients. For the caloric test, he typically used only cold water because he found that hot water was disagreeable to most patients. He did occasionally use hot water, however, particularly if he required a strong stimulus to reverse a spontaneous nystagmus (nystagmus that was already present without any stimulation).

For his rotational test, Bárány seated the patient on a swivel chair and manually rotated the patient 10 times in 20 seconds and then suddenly stopped with the patient facing him (Figure 11.1). He measured the duration of post-rotatory nystagmus in each direction immediately after the chair was stopped. He found that normal subjects had an average duration of post-rotatory nystagmus of approximately 22 seconds, although there was a good deal of inter-subject variability. Much of this variability could be traced to the difficulty in manually maintaining a constant velocity and then producing a uniform sudden deceleration. Furthermore, the response to the initial acceleration was often not completed before the deceleration began, resulting in interaction between the two responses. Bárány found that patients with one-sided inner ear damage typically had asymmetric post-rotatory nystagmus with stronger nystagmus beating toward the good ear. He explained this on the basis of Ewald's second law: Ampullopetal endolymph flow in the horizontal

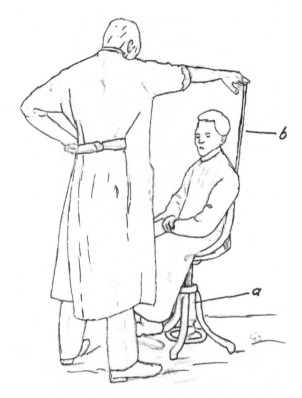

Figure 11.1 BARANY'S ROTATIONAL CHAIR TEST. (a) Rotational device and (b) arm to manually rotate the patient. See text for details. Source: From Bárány R. *Physiologie und Pathologie des Bogengangapparates beim Menschen.* Vienna: Deuticke, 1907.

semicircular canal of the intact ear produces stronger nystagmus compared to ampullofugal flow.

Romberg Test

In 1846, German neurologist Maritz Heinrich Romberg noted that patients with a spinal form of syphilis called tabes dorsalis were unable to stand with their feet together with eyes closed (Figure 11.2). He correctly surmised that because these patients had lost proprioceptive sensation from their muscles and joints, they were unable to stand with their feet together when vision was removed. Bárány was the first to emphasize that patients with acute inner ear damage tended to sway and fall toward the damaged side when standing with their feet together and eyes closed (the Romberg test). Bárány concluded that patients fell to the side of acute vestibular damage because of an asymmetry in the "vestibular tone" arriving at the spinal musculature. With chronic lesions, patients

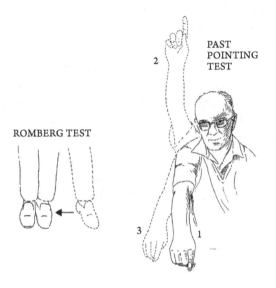

Figure 11.2 SCHEMATIC ILLUSTRATION OF THE ROMBERG TEST AND PAST-POINTING TEST. Source: From Baloh RW, Honrubia V. *Clinical Neurophysiology of the Vestibular System.* 3rd ed. New York: Oxford University Press, 2001.

often fell toward the intact side, which Bárány attributed to the brain's attempt to compensate for the acute vestibular imbalance.

Past-Pointing Test

Bárány devised an elaborate series of tests to measure the phenomenon of past-pointing—a reactive deviation of the extremities often caused by an imbalance in vestibular tone. In 1910, Bárány published a review of pointing deviation and emphasized the importance of having patients sit with their eyes closed to avoid confusion with other orienting information. He systematically evaluated pointing about the shoulder and about the wrist. He performed the test by having the patient place the extended index finger on his own finger, raise the extended arm and index finger to a vertical position, and attempt to return the index finger to his finger (see Figure 11.2). Consistent deviation to one side was defined as past-pointing. Bárány showed that caloric and rotational stimulation consistently induced past-pointing in the direction of the slow phase of induced nystagmus. Similarly, patients with an acutely damaged inner ear past-pointed in the direction of the slow phase of nystagmus. As with the Romberg test, however, Bárány noted that the direction of past-pointing could be in the opposite direction in people with chronic compensated inner ear disorders.

Bárány noted that past-pointing abnormalities were not specific for inner ear damage but also occurred with brain damage. He believed that distinct locations within the cerebellum (the part of the brain that controls balance) controlled pointing accuracy and thereby, by performing a careful past-pointing examination, the neurologist could localize a lesion within the cerebellum (Bárány, 1912). He became interested in the phenomenon when he noted that patients with one-sided cerebellar tumors showed a past-pointing reaction in the extremities on the side of the tumor only. He believed that if he had enough patients with localized cerebellar tumors, he might be able to identify the cerebellar past-pointing centers. Unfortunately, more recent studies have found past-pointing test results to be too inconsistent and unreliable to be of much use in the routine neurological examination.

Bárány's Syndrome

The overall cavalier attitude of surgeons at the time is illustrated by Bárány's description of a new clinical syndrome that he called "Bárány's syndrome" (Bárány, 1912). The syndrome consisted of episodes of vertigo, fluctuating hearing loss, occipital headaches, and a spontaneous outward past-pointing error. Bárány concluded that the syndrome was probably related to migraine because most patients had migraine headaches for many years and many patients had relatives with migraine. The mechanism was "either a temporary swelling or swollen condition of the cerebellar hemisphere, or more likely an abnormal liquid secretion, a liquid collection on the outer side of the cerebellum" (p. 83). With this in mind, Bárány proceeded to operate on a patient with this syndrome with the goal of relieving pressure on the cerebellum. He reported that immediately after the operation, the headache and vomiting ceased only to have the headache occur on the other side, and while the hearing on the operated side returned to normal, the other ear became noticeably deaf. Bárány then noted the pointing error outward on the other side. He therefore operated on the second side. Again, the headache stopped and the past-pointing error disappeared. Bárány concluded that "these cases with inner ear lesions, headache in the occiput, dizziness and pointing error outward for the wrist joint, that is in cases with Bárány's syndrome, must be amenable to an early operative therapy" (p. 87). In retrospect, these patients of Bárány probably had basilar migraine, a condition in which occipital headache, episodic vertigo, and fluctuating hearing can occur. Spontaneous remissions are common, and placebo effects (in this case surgery) can be dramatic. One can only assume that Barany's findings on his past-pointing tests were spurious because they defy any logical interpretation (in the realm of wishful thinking).

First Description of Benign Paroxysmal Positional Vertigo

During his lifetime, Bárány published more than 200 scientific articles in the field of otolaryngology. Most of his innovative work on the vestibular system was published prior to his move to Uppsala, Sweden, after the war. In Uppsala, he described several new surgical techniques, including an operation to produce a fistula in the wall of the horizontal semicircular canal to improve hearing in patients with otosclerosis. He later abandoned this technique, however, because the fistula invariably closed and the hearing loss returned. Probably his most important article published while he lived in Uppsala was a short paper in *Acta Otolaryngologica* in 1921 describing a young woman with positional vertigo and nystagmus (Bárány, 1921). This was the summary of a lecture to the Society of Physicians in Stockholm, October 12, 1920. His assistant, Dr. Karlefors, showed him a 27-year-old woman who developed vertigo every time she lay on her right side. Her only other symptom was recurrent headaches during the past year. When Bárány turned her onto her right side, she developed (as translated in Lanska and Remler, 1997)

> a strong rotatory (torsional) nystagmus to the right with a vertical component upwards, which when looking to the right was purely rotatory, and when looking to the left was purely vertical [Figure 11.3]. The attack lasted about a half-minute, and was accompanied by severe vertigo and nausea. If, immediately after the end of an attack, the head was again turned to the right, no attack occurred. The patient had to lie for some time on her back or on her left side in order to evoke a new attack. (p. 1168)

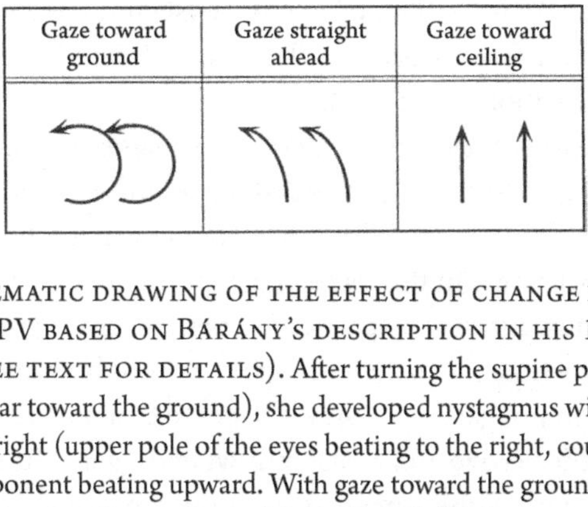

Gaze toward ground	Gaze straight ahead	Gaze toward ceiling

Figure 11.3 SCHEMATIC DRAWING OF THE EFFECT OF CHANGE IN GAZE POSITION ON BPPV BASED ON BÁRÁNY'S DESCRIPTION IN HIS 1921 PUBLICATION (SEE TEXT FOR DETAILS). After turning the supine patient's head to the right (right ear toward the ground), she developed nystagmus with a torsional component to the right (upper pole of the eyes beating to the right, counterclockwise) and a vertical component beating upward. With gaze toward the ground (right), the nystagmus was torsional; with gaze toward the ceiling (left), the nystagmus was vertical.

Her hearing was normal, and both her general and neurologic examinations were normal. She also showed normal caloric reactions in both ears.

Bárány had written about positional nystagmus on several prior occasions and had described a similar rotatory nystagmus triggered by head position changes that he had assumed resulted from damage to the semicircular canals (Bárány, 1910). However, in this case, he conducted a series of experiments with the patient that convinced him that the positional nystagmus was originating from the otolith organs (the macules) rather than the semicircular canals (Bárány, 1921). He reasoned that if the nystagmus originated from a semicircular canal, then it would occur with movement in the plane of that canal regardless of the beginning and ending position. He began his examination with the patient lying on her left side with her left cheek resting on a pillow. Bárány described his experiment as follows (as translated in Lanska and Remler, 1997):

> When I moved her head to the right, but only so far that she assumed a supine position, there occurred no vertigo and no nystagmus, even if the time after an attack had been very long. In contrast, nystagmus occurred immediately in the supine position when the patient turned her head just a little bit to the right. It could therefore be shown that the identical movement did not produce riystagmus when the movement was from the left side position to the middle position, but produced severe nystagmus when, through the same movement, she came to lay on her right side. If the position and not the movement caused the vertigo, then it would be irrelevant in which way the vertigo position was reached. (p. 1169)

Bárány then had the patient sit up and tilt her head first onto her left shoulder and then, after returning to the upright position, onto her right shoulder. Again, she had no nystagmus with her head to the left or on returning to the upright position, but she immediately developed vertigo and nystagmus with her head tilted to the right. Bárány concluded that the nystagmus and vertigo must originate from the otolith organs because they are activated by the position of the head rather than rotation of the head.

Bárány was well aware that the semicircular canals sense angular acceleration and are unresponsive to gravity, whereas the otolith organs respond to linear acceleration including gravity. With a few simple experiments, he established that identical movements in the same plane with different starting and ending positions resulted in different responses (sometimes nystagmus and sometimes not). However, any time the patient brought her head back and to the right, this resulted in nystagmus regardless of how she got to that position. The logical conclusion was that the vertigo and nystagmus were triggered from stimulating the gravity-sensing organs of the inner ears, the otolith organs.

As discussed in Chapter 17, Bárány was wrong in this conclusion, but he did provide the first unequivocal description of benign paroxysmal positional nystagmus. He identified the two key features of the nystagmus—the torsional and vertical components that changed with the eye position in the orbit and the fatigue with repeated positioning (decreased response when he repeated the positioning). Bárány induced the positional nystagmus by turning the head to the side while the patient was lying supine or turning the head back and to the side while the patient was seated. He failed to recognize that the speed of the positioning was important for inducing the nystagmus. Bárány mentioned nothing about the patient's clinical course or outcome. As we now know, benign paroxysmal positional vertigo (BPPV) is relatively uncommon in patients younger than age 30 years; it is most common in patients older than age 60 years. When seen in a young patient such as described by Bárány, it is often preceded by head trauma, ear infection, or in association with migraine. How migraine predisposes to development of BPPV at a young age is unclear. The fact that Bárány's patient experienced recurrent headaches raises the likelihood that this first clearly described case of BPPV was associated with migraine.

Bárány was well aware that there were problems with his conclusion that the positional vertigo and nystagmus resulted from damage to the gravity-sensing otolith organs. It was generally believed that nystagmus could only originate from stimulation of the semicircular canals. Based on the work of Magnus (1924) and de Kleyn (1922), the otolith organs were thought to participate in tonic reflexes such as sustained eye deviation with head tilt, whereas the semicircular canals generated dynamic reflexes such as nystagmus. However, the prominent torsional movements of the eyes in his patient with positional nystagmus reminded Bárány of the ocular counter-rolling movements that occur in normal human subjects when they are tilted to the side. He had studied ocular counter-rolling in 1906 and even developed a special apparatus to induce and measure the torsional eye movements (Bárány, 1907). Bárány had initially assumed that the counter-rolling eye movements originated from the vertical semicircular canals, but he now believed that they might be mediated through the otolith organs.

In 1909, Karl Wittmaack noted that he could dislodge the heavy otolithic membrane from the otolith organs of guinea pigs by rotating them at high speeds in a centrifuge (2000 rpm). On histologic preparations of the guinea pigs' inner ears, Wittmaack noted pieces of otolithic membrane (otoconia) throughout the membranous labyrinth far from their normal location on the receptor epithelium overlying the afferent nerve terminals (the macule). Magnus and de Kleyn (1926) repeated these experiments and tested eye movements in guinea pigs after the otoconia was dislodged from the macules. They found that static compensatory eye movements to tilt, ocular counter-rolling, disappeared. In his

1921 paper, Bárány suggested that measurement of counter-rolling eye movements associated with head tilt might be a simple test of otolith function in human patients. Breuer and Kreidl had already measured counter-rolling eye movements in human subjects during centrifugal acceleration in 1898 (see Chapter 4). One must keep in mind, however, that these counter-rolling eye movements generated by otolith stimulation were tonic movements and not nystagmus. The issue of whether nystagmus could originate from a damaged otolith organ continued to be at the center of the controversy regarding the mechanism of BPPV throughout much of the 20th century.

Bárány concluded his 1921 paper on positional nystagmus by briefly mentioning that he had described a patient with a central type of positional nystagmus in 1913 that was distinctly different from the nystagmus of the patient he described in 1921. His earlier patient had multiple sclerosis, and she developed a horizontal nystagmus every time she would lie on her left side. Contrary to the patient with BPPV, the positional nystagmus in the patient with multiple sclerosis did not stop after half a minute but continued as long as the patient lay on that side.

References

Bárány R. *Physiologie und Pathologie des Bogengangapparates beim Menschen.* Vienna: Deuticke, 1907.

Bárány R. Neue Untersuchungsmethoden, die Beziehungen zwischen Vestibularapparat, Kleinhirn, Grosshirn und Rückenmark betreffend. *Wien Med Wochenschr* 1910;60:2033.

Bárány R (DeSwarte LT, trans). The vestibular apparatus and the central nervous system. *Laryngoscope* 1912;2:81–89.

Bárány R. Diagnose von Krankheitserscheinungen im Bereiche des Otolithenapparates. *Acta Otolaryngol* 1921;2:434–437.

de Kleyn A. Recherches quantitatives sur les positions compensatories l'oeil chez de lapin. *Arch Need Physiol* 1922;7:138.

Lanska DJ, Remler B. Benign paroxysmal positional vertigo: Classic descriptions, origins of the provocative positioning technique, and conceptual developments. *Neurology* 1997;48:1167–1177.

Magnus R. *Körperstellung.* Berlin: Springer-Verlag, 1924.

Magnus R, de Kleyn A. Funktion des Bogengange—und Otolithenapparates bei Säugern. In *Handb d Norm u Pathol Physiol Bd* 11, S 868–908. Berlin: Springer, 1926.

Wittmaack K. Über Veränderungen im inneren Ohre nach Rotationen. *Verh Dtsch Ges Otol* 1909;18:150.

12

Bárány's Life in Uppsala and His Work with Lorente de Nó

Despite being a Nobel laureate, Robert Bárány lived a quiet, even lonely, existence in Uppsala, Sweden (a quiet, sleepy university town approximately 2 hours north of Stockholm by train) after the war (Holmgren, 1936). All of his energies went into developing and maintaining a new otolaryngological clinic at the university. His days were spent examining patients and performing surgery, and his evenings were spent reading scientific books and journals. He lived in an apartment with his wife and three children, rarely venturing out into the town in the evenings. Carl Olav Nylen (1965), who served as an assistant to Bárány in 1919 and 1920, described Bárány as

> outwardly self-absorbed, silent and thoughtful [but] the moment the "standard of science" was raised, Bárány became fired by the flame of enthusiasm. His capacity for work and study was prodigious, so that at times he would read and write day and night with little rest. (p. 318)

Bárány had relatively little interest in the arts, although he liked music and, according to Nylen (1965), he played the piano well, being particularly fond of Schumann. He was an enthusiastic outdoors man and, despite his ankylosed knee, enjoyed long hikes and mountain climbing, and he regularly played tennis, often with his assistant Nylen. Being a Nobel laureate, Bárány had frequent visitors to his clinic from all around the world, and Nylen commented, "he was unstinting in his efforts to instruct and satisfy their desire for knowledge" (p. 318). Nylen himself went on to a productive career in neurotology with a particular interest in the classification of positional nystagmus.

The Bárány family had a great deal of difficulty adjusting to their new life in Uppsala. Bárány's wife in particular had difficulty with the Swedish language and customs. She believed that Uppsala lacked culture and could not be compared to her beloved Vienna. The family typically returned to Austria each year for their vacation. The children saw little of their father because of his long hours at the hospital and clinic. Bárány typically returned home for lunch each day followed by a nap during which the children had to maintain complete silence. As the boys grew older, they were able to spend more time with their father, typically having at least one tennis match with him each week. After Ernst decided on a career in medicine, he and his father became much closer, often spending hours discussing material that Ernst was studying.

An incident that further illustrates Bárány's personality and his relationship with his children occurred while the family was on vacation in Gotland in 1924 (Joas, 1997). Earlier that year, Franz had injured his nose while playing soccer, leaving him with a severe septal deviation. Bárány decided that the vacation was the ideal time to repair the deviation. On a hot, humid August day, he took Franz to the local hospital despite Franz's plans to enter a tennis tournament that day. Bárány used cocaine for a local anesthesia and proceeded with the operation despite the fact that Franz briefly lost consciousness and then continuously screamed. Bárány, in turn, complained about the poor quality of the equipment in the small operating room that he was provided.

Lorente de Nó (1987), who arrived in Uppsala in 1924 to work with Bárány, described how Bárány spent much of his time living within himself:

> He could remain silent and oblivious to the outside world for considerable lengths of time, while intensely thinking about some scientific problem. While at home he sometimes fell into such trances when he was in the middle of a conversation probably because something that had just been said had set his thinking mechanism into motion. Those trances always ended in the same manner. Without saying a word, Bárány took out of his coat pocket a pencil and an oversized notebook and making use of his mastery in stenography he rapidly recorded sequences of thought that otherwise might have been forgotten and lost. (p. 8)

Bárány not infrequently would awaken during the night and begin recording some thoughts that were going through his mind. He was never bothered by the lack of sleep because he was able to take short naps throughout the day. Lorente marveled,

> He could go to sleep at will, for the length of time prescribed by him in advance. On a number of occasions during our lengthy conversations he would become physically tired. When this happened Bárány would say to me "Let me sleep for ten or twenty minutes" or for whatever number of minutes he felt he needed. After the prescribed time

Bárány awoke and resumed the conversation precisely at the point of interruption. (p. 8)

Lorente also noted that Bárány frequently took his timed naps during scientific meetings if the material was less than stimulating.

Bárány was extraordinarily intelligent but rather naive, according to Lorente (1987). Bárány's passion was to acquire knowledge and to understand how the human body works. Lorente noted that "he strongly disliked jokes, banalities and unfounded statements and he hated illogical conclusions" (p. 8). Like Josef Breuer, he was known to sharply rebuke colleagues who made illogical statements or showed poor judgment. Unlike Breuer, however, he lacked the social skills to make these comments without creating a personal enemy. Bárány was considered proud and conceited.

The Brain and the Neuronal Theory

When Rafael Lorente de Nó came to Uppsala in 1924 to work with Bárány, his main goal was to study the central nervous system pathways of the vestibular nystagmus response. In Bárány's 1907 landmark book on the physiology and pathology of the vestibular system, he described a patient with a lesion involving the reticular formation of the pons close to the abducens nucleus who could only generate the slow phase of nystagmus, not the fast phase (Figure 12.1). With caloric or rotational stimulation, the patient's eyes slowly deviated to one side and became pinned, unable to generate the quick corrective components. The patient also had a complete loss of voluntary eye movements. Based on this case, Bárány concluded that there must be separate centers in the brainstem for the production of the slow and fast phases of nystagmus. He further speculated that the center for generating fast phases was in the reticular substance next to the abducens nucleus (where the lesion was located in his patient) and that this quick component was under the influence of cortical control. Somehow, the cerebral cortex monitored the slow phase deviation and regularly interrupted it with quick resetting movements by activating the quick component center in the reticular substance.

Before discussing the central connections of the vestibulo-ocular pathways in more detail, it is useful to consider the overall state of knowledge regarding the anatomy and physiology of the central nervous system at the turn of the 20th century (Katz-Sidlow, 1998). The "reticular theory" championed by the German anatomist Josef von Gerlach and solidified by the Italian anatomist Camilo Golgi was the dominant theory of how the brain worked, although the "neuronal theory" of Ramon y Cajal was rapidly replacing it. Gerlach contended that the

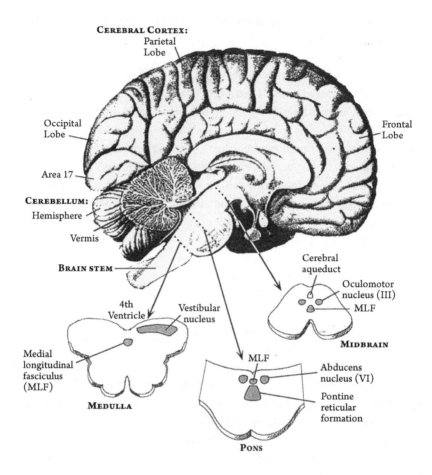

Figure 12.1 SCHEMATIC DRAWING OF THE BRAIN WITH PARTICULAR EMPHASIS ON BRAINSTEM CENTERS INVOLVED IN THE VESTIBULO-OCULAR REFLEXES.

nervous system was composed of a network of cells that anastomosed with each other, forming a closed lattice network. Golgi provided support for this reticular theory with his new staining technique that used a chrome silver reaction to show the diffuse interstitial network of nerve fibers. Golgi considered the neuronal dendrites to be important for nutrition of the neurons (nerve cells) but not a part of the electrical conducting system. Overall, the reticular theory seemed to unify and simplify the process of signal transmission within the nervous system.

Santiago Ramon y Cajal, a Spanish histologist working independently in Madrid, first came across slides of brain tissue stained with Golgi's chrome silver reaction in 1887 (Cajal, 1966). He was immediately enthralled with the powers of this staining technique; in addition, he made the key discovery that if the technique was used on embryological material before the nerve fibers were myelinated, he could obtain an even clearer picture of the neuronal structure. To Cajal's amazement, he found that the terminal ramifications of every nerve fiber ended freely, not in a diffuse network as maintained by Gerlach and Golgi. Cajal thus developed the independent neuronal theory based on the idea that nerve fibers terminate next to the cell bodies and dendrites of other nerve cells and that, because there is no continuity between the nerve cells, nerve impulses must be transmitted across the contacts. The German anatomist Heinrich Wilhelm Gotfried von Waldeyer was the first to use the term *neuron* to describe the "nervous unit" (Katz-Sidlow, 1998).

In the early 20th century, Cajal's hypothesis was supported by overwhelming evidence, particularly by studies in invertebrates, in which nerve cells are easier to see. It was a remarkable irony that Golgi's staining technique allowed Cajal to develop proof that the reticular theory championed by Golgi was incorrect. Golgi was not easily swayed by facts, however, and a heated debate raged between the two men right up until they jointly received the Nobel Prize in 1906. Golgi refused to give in even at the Nobel lecture. Despite the overwhelming data supporting the new neuronal theory, he argued that his own studies proved "the anatomical and functional continuity between nerve cells. And that is the reason why I have not been able to accept the idea of this independence of each nerve cell" (Golgi, 1967, p. 201).

Lorente had worked with Ramon y Cajal in Madrid for 4 years and was highly proficient in performing the Golgi silver staining technique. In Uppsala, Bárány promised to supply the laboratory equipment necessary for stimulating the peripheral vestibular receptors and for recording the eye muscle responses— equipment that was not available in Madrid.

Lorente de Nó and Bárány in Spain

Lorente first met Bárány in December 1923 when Bárány was invited to Lorente's home town of Zaragoza, Spain, to give a series of lectures (Lorente de Nó, 1987). Lorente had already been working in Cajal's laboratory for more than 3 years and had a particular interest in the vestibular neural pathways. Lorente approached Bárány after the first lecture, and they began the first of several prolonged discussions that went well into the night. Bárány was particularly interested in Lorente's Golgi stains of the cerebral cortex because Lorente's work contained details that seemed to conflict with what Bárány had been reading in the literature. At that time, Bárány was just beginning to work on his "general theory of the cerebral cortex," so he found Lorente's detailed histology very exciting. On the other hand, Lorente was fascinated by Bárány's clinical observations in patients with vestibular deficits, particularly his patient with the absent fast components after a pontine lesion. Bárány had noted at autopsy that the lesion in the pons involved the reticular formation well below the surface. In his experiments with rabbits, Lorente was able to remove fast components of nystagmus by making a short, narrow incision along the midline of the medulla and pons (see Figure 12.1), thus interrupting the connections between the two sides but leaving the connections from the inner ear to the abducens nucleus on the same side intact (Lorente de Nó, 1933). Lorente went on to show Bárány his rabbit experiment, and Bárány suggested a series of other experiments that could be performed to elucidate the central mechanism of vestibular nystagmus. He suggested that Lorente stimulate the semicircular canals of rabbits by rotation while at the same time recording the responses of the individual eye muscles. Because the equipment for such experiments was not available in Madrid at the time, Bárány suggested that Lorente come to Uppsala, where he could provide Lorente with the necessary equipment to carry out his experiments. This was an exciting offer for Lorente, but he noted that because of the military conscription in Spain, he was scheduled to start his military service within a few weeks and, in addition, he did not have the funds to travel and work in Uppsala. These seemed minor detriments to Bárány because he responded, "Now am I sure you are coming to Uppsala because I know that your problems can easily be solved" (Lorente de Nó, 1987, p. 6).

Following Bárány's lecture series, he and Lorente traveled to Madrid, where Bárány visited with Cajal and pointed out the important scientific achievements to be obtained if Lorente were to work with him for several years in Uppsala. Cajal was wholly supportive of the visit to Uppsala because he strongly believed that young Spanish scientists should work in foreign laboratories. Bárány was well aware of the prestige that Nobel laureates enjoyed in Spain at that time, so he was convinced that if two Nobel laureates—he and Cajal—made a request to the head of the Spanish government, the request would be honored. The next day, Cajal and Bárány visited with the appropriate government officials, and it was immediately decided that Lorente's military service could be postponed indefinitely and he was granted a government salary that would allow him to "live comfortably" in Sweden.

Before Bárány left Spain, Lorente accompanied him on a visit to Toledo, a mandatory visit for any tourist visiting Madrid (Lorente de Nó, 1987). This beautiful city known for its remarkable art treasures is a short train ride from Madrid, permitting a single-day visit with the morning train arriving at approximately 10:00 a.m. and the afternoon train leaving at approximately 5:00 p.m. Lorente's description of Barany's visit to Toledo says much about Bárány's personality and his lack of interest in the arts. Lorente noted,

We first went into the magnificent cathedral but as soon as he had taken two steps inside the door Bárány looked around and said: "Ah!

A church! I have seen churches before!" whereupon he turned around and walked to the street. Thinking that religious buildings had no interest for him, we took him to the El Greco museum. Right after entering there, Bárány said "Ah! A collection of artistic reproductions!" and he turned around and left. We did not dare to take Bárány to the small church that contains El Greco's famous painting of the Conde de Orgaz, but we believed that we should show him at least one of the two famous synagogues that are among the most beautiful in the world. This time Bárány did not even cross the door. Looking from the outside Bárány repeated his now standard comment: "I have seen synagogues before!" (p. 7)

Giving up on the artistic treasures, they decided to have an early lunch and take a walk through the beautiful surroundings of Toledo since Bárány was so fond of hiking. However, because of persistent rain, they ended up playing billiards for the remainder of the afternoon until the return train left for Madrid.

Lorente de Nó Works on Central Vestibular Pathways with Bárány

When Lorente arrived in Uppsala in 1924 to work with Bárány, he had already formulated several basic concepts regarding the central vestibulo-ocular connections based on his familiarity with Cajal's work and his own use of the Golgi silver stain on neuronal histological sections. The simplest concept of the semicircular canal oculomotor connection was a three-neuronal arc. The first neuron senses the endolymph movement in the semicircular canal with its afferent terminal and carries the signal into the brainstem vestibular nuclei, where it transmits it to a second neuron whose cell body rests within the nucleus. The second neuron, through its axon, transmits the signal to a third neuron, an oculomotor neuron. The motor neuron activates an eye muscle and produces the appropriate eye movement. This suggests a simple wiring diagram of connecting the appropriate neurons originating in each of the three semicircular canals with the six oculomotor nuclei that control the six eye muscles that turn the globe. However, based on his and Cajal's detailed histological studies, Lorente was aware that neuronal connections were much more complex than such a simple wiring diagram (Lorente de Nó, 1933). All the neurons that they studied connected with neurons in multiple different centers (the law of plurality of connections), and all the neurons gave off collaterals that either fed back to neurons that were connected to them or to interneurons that fed back to these neurons (the law of reciprocity of connections). These anatomical features suggested that the central vestibulo-ocular pathways were much more complex than a simple direct forward passage of signals from one neuron to another.

Dating back to the work of Breuer, it had generally been assumed that the two components of nystagmus, the slow and fast components, were fundamentally different in nature, each generated by a different neuronal center. Bárány assumed that the center for fast component production required cortical control. However, Lorente's lesion experiments in rabbits showed that nystagmus could still be generated after the entire cerebral cortex was removed or after cuts above and below the region of the vestibular nuclei. All these findings led Lorente to conclude that the nystagmus triggered by stimulating the semicircular canals was an alternating reflex, no different from other rhythmic reflexes such as the scratch reflex triggered by stimulating the skin.

For his studies of the vestibulo-ocular reflex in Uppsala, Lorente chose the animal with which he was most familiar, the rabbit, because this animal's eye movements are almost exclusively driven by the vestibular system. He operated on the animals under ether anesthesia, but because the vestibular reflexes disappeared during anesthesia, he removed the cerebral cortex so that the animals' reflexes could be studied when they were awake but they could feel no pain (Lorente de Nó, 1932). The reflex reactions of all six ocular muscles were recorded by connecting the individual ocular muscles with isotonic levers that were recorded simultaneously on an 18-inch drum. These isotonic recordings offered a permanent record of the existence and direction of nystagmus and also slow tonic contractions when fast components were not present. To excite the semicircular canals, Lorente used both rotations in the plane of the canal and also a caloric stimulus that he generated by touching the bony canals with a cold or warm needle. This latter technique allowed him to cause ampullopetal and ampullofugal endolymph flow sequentially in a single semicircular canal. As Breuer had previously observed, Lorente noted that when the hot and cold needle was brought in contact with the canal, after a short latent period, a nystagmus arose that increased in intensity to a certain maximum depending on the temperature of the needle and remained relatively constant as long as the needle was resting on the canal (Lorente de Nó, 1932, 1933). When the needle was removed, the nystagmus in the plane of the stimulated canal remained for a certain time (after-discharge), which Lorente attributed to two processes: (1) the time necessary for the bony canal to recover to body temperature and (2) a central after-discharge within the central vestibulo-ocular pathways (now called velocity storage).

For his brainstem lesion experiments around the vestibular nuclei, Lorente first removed the cerebellar midline that, if removed completely, did not result in any spontaneous nystagmus. He then proceeded to make systematic lesions in different locations around the vestibular nuclei and recorded the effect on the induced semicircular canal ocular reflexes. From a series of experiments using this experimental model, Lorente made several basic conclusions about the vestibulo-ocular reflex pathways (Figure 12.2). First, the neurons within the vestibulo-ocular pathways are always in a state of "automatic activity" that is chiefly generated in the inner ear although still partially remains even after extirpation of the inner ear. Second, the neurons within the vestibulo-ocular pathways form closed circuits that he called "self-reexciting chains," which are capable of rhythmic activity and which can explain the prolonged after-discharge. Third, numerous pathways between the vestibular nuclei and the motoneurons are always being used at the same time so that the reflex reactions are not determined by one nucleus but, rather, are the consequence of the interaction of all the nuclei and the paths of the whole vestibular system.

These experiments by Lorente provide the framework for our current understanding of the role of the inner ear and the brainstem in generating semicircular canal-ocular reflex responses (nystagmus). If a rabbit or a person is rotated at a constant velocity and suddenly stopped, the after-nystagmus is maximum immediately and then gradually decays exponentially with a time constant defined as the time it takes the slow phase velocity of the nystagmus to decay to 63% of the initial maximum value. It can be shown that the time constant of the canal-ocular reflex (T_{cor}) is made up of two components—the time constant of the cupulo-endolymph system acting as a damped pendulum and the time constant

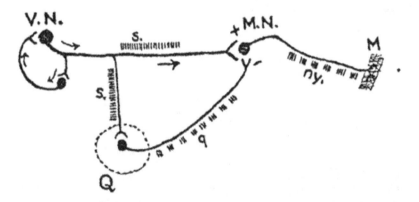

Figure 12.2 Lorente de Nó's schematic drawing of the vestibulo-ocular reflex. The signal sensed by the afferent nerve is carried to the vestibular nucleus (V.N.), where the signal in turn is passed on to the motor neurons (M.N.), which activate the appropriate eye muscles (M). He also illustrates the reverberating circuits within the vestibular nucleus (with a feedback neuron) and an additional center located in the pontine reticular formation (Q) that generates the fast components of nystagmus. The slow component signal (s.) is passed directly on to the motor neurons and also is passed on to the pontine reticular formation, where it activates neurons that generate the fast component (q). Source: From Lorente de Nó, R. Vestibulo-ocular reflexes. *Arch Neurol Psychiat* 1933;30:245.

of the central feedback pathways described by Lorente (Figure 12.3). The time constant of the cupula-endolymph system (often called T_1) depends on the viscosity of the endolymph and the elasticity of the cupula, and it is estimated to be 5–7 seconds. By contrast, T_{cor} for the horizontal semicircular canal-ocular reflex is approximately three times longer due to velocity storage in the central feedback pathways described by Lorente. In other words, after a sudden stop with rotation in the horizontal plane, the nystagmus lasts approximately three times longer than it takes for the cupula to return to its resting position. Interestingly, there is relatively little velocity storage in the vertical canal-ocular reflexes so that T_1 and T_{cor} are approximately the same. As discussed later, this explains why benign paroxysmal positional vertigo episodes associated with the horizontal canal variant last longer than episodes with the more common posterior canal variant.

Lorente conducted experiments on the central mechanisms of the vestibular eye reflexes from 1924 to 1927, working in the laboratory that Bárány provided him in Uppsala. Lorente recalled that a few weeks after he arrived in Uppsala in 1924, he decided to pay a visit to the Báránys after having dinner at a nearby restaurant (Lorente de Nó, 1987). Bárány was extremely pleased to see him, and they had a lively productive 2-hour conversation. Bárány urged him to return the next evening, and during the next several years, their 2-hour after-dinner conversation in which they discussed both scientific and social issues became an almost nightly ritual. Bárány regularly critiqued Lorente's experiments on the vestibular eye reflexes and quizzed Lorente on his extensive knowledge of the morphology and connections of cortical neurons.

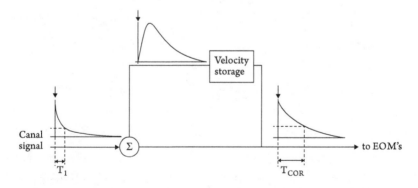

Figure 12.3 PROLONGATION OF THE TIME CONSTANT OF THE CANAL OCULAR REFLEX (TCOR) BY VELOCITY STORAGE IN THE FEEDBACK PATHWAYS DESCRIBED BY LORENTE DE NÓ. A step change in angular velocity occurred at time 0 (vertical arrow). T_1 represents the time constant of the cupula–endolymph system measured from the average response of primary afferent neurons. Source: From Baloh RW, Honrubia V. *Clinical Neurophysiology of the Vestibular System.* 3rd ed. New York: Oxford University Press, 2001.

At approximately this time, Bárány was losing interest in his clinical work and was devoting most of his time developing a new general theory on the function of the cerebral cortex. This is somewhat amazing because Bárány had little background in either the anatomy or the physiology of the cerebral cortex. During their nightly discussions, Lorente served as the

> interlocutor for Bárány for I would be capable of preventing the making of assumptions that were either too simple or too complicated and also capable of invalidating explanations that either conflicted with known facts or were based on the postulate of arrangements of doubtful or unknown existence. (Lorente de Nó, 1987, p. 12)

These discussions often became "quite noisy." One area of heated debate was Bárány's pet theory that the two granular layers of the occipital cortex (area 17) of animals with binocular vision each received input from a different eye (see Figure 12.1). Based on his knowledge of the cerebral cortical anatomy, Lorente believed that this was highly unlikely, but he admitted that the necessary anatomical and physiologic information to prove the point one way or the other did not exist.

Toward the end of 1926, they decided that Lorente should go to Berlin for a few months to work in the Neurobiological Institute of Oscar and Cecil Vogt, where there was a large collection of histological brain slides from numerous different animal species. At approximately the same time, Professor S. E. Heuschen of Stockholm, who also disputed Bárány's theory, visited Berlin to determine what information Lorente was able to discover. When it was clear that they could not answer the question with the material that was available, Lorente suggested to Heuschen that he could settle the question if he had access to the brains of two or three young monkeys so that he could prepare histological sections using Golgi's silver staining technique. Heuschen was so intent on obtaining an answer that he bought three young nemestrinus monkeys with his own money. The Golgi stains that Lorente prepared on these monkey brains strongly suggested that both eyes projected to both granular layers of the occipital cortex, although both agreed that anatomical data alone could not provide a definitive answer.

When Lorente returned to Uppsala from Berlin in January 1927, he told Bárány of his findings on the occipital cortex of the three young monkeys, but Bárány was still not convinced and refused to give up his theory (Lorente de Nó, 1987). Against Lorente's advice, Bárány announced that he would present his theory in a communication to the Swedish Medical Society even though he knew Heuschen would be there to dispute the theory. With the anticipation of a heated debate, the hall of the Society was packed to capacity. Lorente noted, "the reaction of the audience after the end of Heuschen's energetic and devastating speech caused Bárány intense displeasure" (p. 13). That meeting marked the end of Bárány's work on the theory of the cerebral cortex.

Bárány's Final Years

As a result of Bárány's decreasing interest in clinical practice, the main source of income for his family diminished and their standard of living suffered. When Lorente returned to Uppsala in July 1928 after having been in Spain to fulfill his 10-month military commitment, he became acutely aware of Bárány's financial problems. Lorente (1987) wrote that to reduce the cost of their rent,

> the Báránys had to give up their spacious and comfortable studio-living room. With the room, they also lost the splendid view of the main university building and its plaza. Their spacious living room had been added to the apartment of some wealthy neighbor and to the Báránys there remained available only a small sitting room of irregular geometry, that could accommodate only a few pieces of small furniture. That sitting room had a large window, but with no other view than the bare wall of the next building. We continued our nightly conversations in the new sitting room but we never made even the slightest remark concerning the change. (p. 15)

It was approximately this time that Bárány first became aware of small zones of hemorrhages next to blood vessels in one of his retinas. Bárány had become interested in Purkinje's method for observation of the blood vessels in the optic fundus of one's own eye. As Purkinje noted, this can be accomplished by anyone by pressing a small flashlight against the side of the closed eyeball, which with change in pressure allows the subject to begin to see the entire network of retinal blood vessels in one's own eye. The hemorrhages that Bárány saw were in the extreme periphery of the retina and did not result in vision impairment but were the harbinger of later hemorrhages that would occur in the brain.

Bárány had been aware that he had hypertension for many years but he did not trust the physicians in Uppsala and eventually he started himself on antihypertensive medications. During a visit to the United States, he was evaluated at the Mayo Clinic, where he was told that he had malignant hypertension. He periodically saw physicians in Austria or Germany, but he did not tell any of his colleagues in Uppsala about his medical problems. Ultimately, he suffered repeated attacks of cerebral hemorrhage that progressively impaired his speech and the use of his hands.

Despite these deficits, he continued to read and attempted to write scientific papers using one finger on a typewriter. In a brief biographical sketch on Bárány published in the *Annals of Otology, Rhinology and Laryngology* soon after his death, Bárány's Swedish colleague, Gunnar Holmgren (1936), commented on Bárány's lonely existence after being exiled to Uppsala:

> Transplanted, as he was, to surroundings which for him were strange, far from his home, family and all old friends, and with the comparative isolation which follows transportation from the center to a periphery, he retired to himself and became strange to many amongst his new surroundings. A heavy shadow which long rested on him was a desire for his beloved Vienna, and it was not without bitterness that he contemplated that his own country had not been able to find a place for him. (p. 594)

A large international celebration had been planned for Bárány's 60th birthday on April 22, 1936. Several hundred otologists from throughout the world sent Bárány greetings, and a collection of papers was to be published under Bárány's direction. Unfortunately, he did not live to see his day of honor; he died unexpectedly in Uppsala on April 8. His body was cremated, and he was buried at the Stockholm crematory.

Regarding Bárány's antagonists at the Politzer Vienna Otology Clinic, both Gustav Alexander and Heinrich Neumann went on to have productive academic careers. Alexander had more than 200 publications, most of which focused on the inner ear, particularly on ear infections and their intracranial complications. He is probably best known for his description of the effect of changes in gaze position on spontaneous vestibular nystagmus, now known as Alexander's law. Gaze in the direction of the fast component increases the amplitude of the nystagmus, whereas gaze away from the direction of the fast component decreases the amplitude. Alexander was responsible for starting Austria's first kindergarten for deaf-mutes, and he was a major supporter of an institution for the care of blind deaf-mutes. His life came to a tragic end in 1932 when he was killed by a disgruntled patient. Alexander had operated on the man's nose in 1905 while he was a young assistant in Politzer's clinic. Dissatisfied with the operation, the patient tried to sue Alexander, and when this failed he attempted to shoot Alexander but again failed. After a stay in a psychiatric hospital, he left Austria only to return in 1932, at which time he successfully shot Alexander (Majer and Kopec, 1985).

Heinrich Neumann became known for his surgical skills and his international clientele. He became head of the Vienna Otology Clinic after Politzer retired. The kings of Spain, Romania, and England were among his patients.

When Austria was occupied by German troops in 1938, Neumann was arrested because of his Jewish ancestry but was set free through the intervention of the Duke of Windsor. Neumann spent the next year and a half traveling abroad raising money for emigration of fellow Jews. The author Hans Habe used Neumann as the central character for his novel *The Mission*, which was based on Neumann's participation in the refugee conference in Evian organized by President Roosevelt. Neumann died in New York in 1939 (Majer and Kopec, 1985).

References

Bárány R. *Physiologie und Pathologie des Bogengangapparates beim Menschen.* Vienna: Deuticke, 1907.

Cajal S (Craigie EH, Cano J, trans). *Recollections of My Life: Santiago Ramon y Cajal.* Cambridge, MA: MIT Press, 1966.

Golgi C. Neuron doctrine—Theory and facts. In: *Nobel Lectures: Physiology or Medicine.* New York: Elsevier, 1967, pp 201–202.

Holmgren G. Robert Barany: 1876–1936. *Ann Otol Rhinol Laryngol* 1936;45:593–595.

Joas G. *Robert Bárány (1876–1936): Leben und Werk.* Frankfurt am Main: Lang, 1997.

Katz-Sidlow RJ. The formulation of the neuron doctrine: The island of Cajal. *Arch Neurol* 1998;55:237–240.

Lorente de Nó R. The regulation of eye positions and movements induced by the labyrinth. *Laryngoscope* 1932;42:233.

Lorente de Nó R. Vestibulo-ocular reflex arc. *Arch Neurol Psychiatr* 1933;30:245–291.

Lorente de Nó R. Facets of the life and work of Professor Robert Barany (1876–1936). In: *Vestibular System.* Graham MD, Kemink JL, eds. New York: Raven Press, 1987, pp 1–16.

Majer EH, S Kopec M. *History of Oto-rhino-laryngology in Austria. An Illustrated Document.* Vienna: Verlag Christian Brandstätter, 1985.

Nylen CO. Robert Barany. *Arch Otolaryngol* 1965;82:316–319.

CHARLES HALLPIKE (1900–1979)

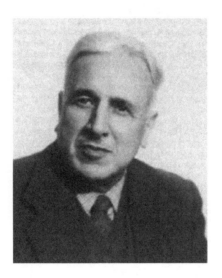

Although scientific medicine became the dominant model for medical education in the first half of the 20th century, the day-to-day practice of medicine lagged far behind. Quackery was still widely prevalent. The balance function of the inner ear was well known due to the work of Breuer and Bárány, but little was known about diseases of the inner ear or how to treat them. Techniques to prepare the inner ear for microscopic examination were finally developed in the early 1900s, and this provided a springboard for the career of Charles Hallpike, who described the pathology of Ménière's disease in 1938. Hallpike went on to describe many common inner ear disorders, including the clinical features and pathology of benign paroxysmal positional vertigo. Throughout his career, Hallpike dealt with the physical disability associated with Legg–Perthes disease and with the perceived stigmata associated with his partial Indian heritage.

13

Hallpike and the Pathology of Ménière's Disease

The clinical practitioners of otology in the first half of the 19th century were mostly quacks (Stevenson and Guthrie, 1949). As Ménière noted, their aggressive treatments often did the patient more harm than good. John Harrison Curtis was a well-known "aurist" in England at the time. Although he had no formal medical training, Curtis had been a dispenser in the Navy and, after marrying well, he set up a private medical practice in the then fashionable Soho Square. With his dynamic personality, he developed a large aristocratic practice including King George IV and the Duke and Duchess of Gloucester. Curtis founded the Dispensary for Diseases of the Ear in 1816 for which he secured Royal patronage. The Dispensary eventually became the Royal Ear Hospital in 1845.

Toynbee and Early Efforts to Study Pathology of the Inner Ear

After hearing Curtis speak at the Medical Society of London in 1837, a young English physician, Joseph Toynbee, vowed to "rescue aural surgery from the hands of quacks" (Weir, 1990, p. 74). In November 1838, Curtis published an article in *Lancet* describing the successful treatment of five patients with deafness by brushing dilute creosote (pitch oil) into the external ear canal (Curtis, 1838a). In keeping with his theory that deafness was caused by impaired production of cerumin, Curtis believed that the creosote improved secretion from the ceruminous glands. Toynbee had enough. He challenged Curtis to "authenticate his cases" in a letter to *Lancet* signed JT (Toynbee, 1838). Curtis responded, "I am much better occupied in attending to the duties of my profession than in replying to the objections of an anonymous writer" (Curtis, 1838b, p. 534).

After another letter from Toynbee and a response from a Curtis supporter, Toynbee (1839) ended his final letter as follows:

> Sir, I must, in common with the medical profession, express my regret that aural surgery is in so degraded a state in this country, that hundreds of deaf persons prefer remaining as they are, to placing themselves under the hands of aurists; and let me assure Mr. Curtis, and the numerous advertising gentlemen of his fraternity, that they, by their ignorance and cupidity, have brought the present odium upon one of the most interesting and important branches of surgery; and that they, instead of "relieving suffering humanity," have produced more misery than any other class of persons now living. To prove the worthlessness of such men; to expose them as a disgrace to society, and to the profession to which they pretend to belong; and, lastly, to endeavor to render aural surgery a scientific pursuit, instead of one calculated to bring discredit upon its followers, shall always continue to be the object of your obedient servant. (p. 734)

Toynbee believed that the only way to develop a rational strategy for the treatment of ear diseases was to dissect the temporal bones of patients with known inner ear diseases. In his classic book, *The Diseases of the Ear* (1860), Toynbee noted that not one dissection of a diseased ear had been done before 1800, although thousands of dissections had been done on most other organs of the body. Toynbee would amass a collection of more than 2000 temporal bone specimens, many of which he obtained as a result of his appointment as aural surgeon to the Asylum for the Deaf and Dumb in Old Kent Road and to the Asylum for Idiots at Earlswood (these were common terms used at the time). The majority of Toynbee's temporal bone specimens were from patients with infections of the middle ear. He was the first to describe a cholesteatoma (overgrowth of tissue triggered by the infection) and a fistula (opening in the bony capsule) of the horizontal semicircular canal, which he noted was a route for infection to spread to the brain. The infection could reach the brain via the cochlear aqueduct, a communicating channel between the perilymph of the inner ear and the fluid surrounding the brain (cerebral spinal fluid). Toynbee came to an untimely death in 1866 at age 51 when he tested a new treatment for tinnitus on himself. He believed that the tinnitus could be cured by inhalation of vapors of hydrocyanic acid and chloroform followed by a Valsalva insufflation.

Wittmaack and His New Technique
for Preparing Temporal Bones

The techniques for examination of the temporal bones developed by Joseph Toynbee were crude by modem-day standards. There were no methods available for fixing the hard and soft tissues of the membranous and bony parts of the inner ear, so the standard histological techniques used to examine other organs were not possible when examining the inner ear. A German otolaryngologist, Karl Philip Ferdinand River Wittmaack, solved these problems and revolutionized the study of temporal bone specimens (Pirsig and Ulrich, 1977).

Wittmaack was born in 1876, the same year as Robert Bárány. After training in multiple different German cities, he began his scientific career at age 28 in Greifswald, Germany. There, he carried out a series of classical experiments on noise damage to the inner ear of guinea pigs. He showed that the damage to the cochlea caused by very loud noise was localized to a circumscribed area of the organ of Corti and spiral ganglia based on the frequency of the noise. In 1908, Wittmaack was appointed professor and head of the Department of Otorhinolaryngology of Jena University in Jena, Germany, where he started his collection of postmortem temporal bone specimens. Wittmaack prepared most of the temporal bone sections by himself, working late into the night after his clinical duties were finished. Wittmaack's biographer, Eckert-Möbius, noted that the curate of Jena University complained that the lights were often burning until midnight on the ground floor of the clinic where Wittmaack's laboratories were situated (Eckert-Möbius, 1972). Wittmaack remarked that he could not prevent himself and his assistants from "exploiting the night for research."

In 1926, Wittmaack moved to a larger clinic in Hamburg, Germany, where he was promised a brand new facility to continue his work on both animal and human temporal bone histology (microscopic anatomy) and to house his large temporal bone collection. He would go on to collect an additional 700 pairs of temporal bones in Hamburg, bringing his overall collection to a total of 1048 pairs of temporal bones. Unfortunately, the promise of a large new facility was broken soon after Wittmaack arrived in Hamburg, with the excuse that a subordinate authority had exceeded its power (Pirsig and Ulrich, 1977). The facility provided to Wittmaack was a small two-story brick building with a few small rooms added in an attached pavilion. In the new pavilion, Wittmaack housed his experimental animals, including monkeys, rabbits, chickens, and guinea pigs, which were adjacent to his histological laboratory, above which the patients' rooms were situated. Wittmaack was noted for his punctilious and volatile personality. He was given the nickname "Rübezahl" (a monster in a Grimm fairy tale) by his colleagues based on his bristly red hair and his frequent mood swings. He began each day by reviewing all of the current cases together with his colleagues and always began his research at exactly 11:00 a.m. Wittmaack carefully documented and maintained detailed records on all the patients from whom he obtained temporal bone specimens.

Although bombing during World War II completely destroyed the main hospital buildings at the University of Hamburg, Wittmaack's temporal bone collections were miraculously saved and even the medical records were preserved. When Wittmaack's home was destroyed by bombs in 1943, he and his wife moved into a section of the surviving hospital for the remainder of the war. In 1946, Wittmaack left his bombed clinic in Hamburg to retire in the mountains of southern Germany at Garmisch-Partenkirchen, two previously separate market towns that were forced to join together by Adolph Hitler prior to their hosting the 1936 winter Olympics. Wittmaack remained bitter and disappointed for the remainder of his life regarding the withdrawn promise for a new clinic at the University of Hamburg (Pirsig and Ulrich, 1977). He never returned to Hamburg after his retirement and remained in total isolation from the German and international otologic community in Garmisch-Partenkirchen, where he died in January 1972.

Worldwide Interest in Wittmaack's Technique

Prior to World War II, physicians from throughout Europe and America flocked to Wittmaack's clinic in Hamburg to learn his technique for studying temporal bone specimens. Wittmaack began with the tedious process of decalcifying the bone with a nitric acid solution that could take up to 6 months. This was followed by a period of dehydration in which the specimens were placed in a series of alcohols of increasing concentration over approximately 10 days. Embedding the tissue in plastic was accomplished by placing the specimens in gradually increasing concentrations of a nitrocellulose preparation over 3 months. After approximately 9 months, a hardened decalcified block of tissue was ready for sectioning with a sharp knife.

A young otologist in London, Charles Skinner Hallpike, became interested in studying temporal bone pathology while he was a research fellow at the Ferens Institute of Otology at the Middlesex Hospital in London in the early 1930s (Whitteridge and Merton, 1984). He had been awarded the Duveen Traveling Studentship in 1930 and a Rockefeller Traveling Fellowship in 1931 allowing him to travel throughout Europe and America to learn the latest developments in otology. He visited the University of Hamburg Ear-Nose and Throat-Clinic, where he learned Wittmaack's method for fixation of the temporal bone. When he returned from his travels, he was awarded a Foulerton Research Fellowship of the Royal Society and set up a temporal bone laboratory at the Ferens Institute.

Hallpike and Cairns Report on the Pathology of Ménière's Syndrome

In December 1934, a 63-year-old dock worker (JB) was referred to the Department of Neurosurgery at the London Hospital to have his vestibular nerve cut because severe attacks of vertigo were making his life unbearable (Hallpike and Cairns, 1938). He had been in good health until 1931, when he began having attacks of vertigo, initially mild and then more severe, causing him to fall to the ground. Because of the increasing frequency and severity of the attacks of vertigo, he could not work for 4 months in 1932 and for 5 months in 1933. As was traditional at the time, JB was treated with Eustachian tube catheterization and sedative drugs, with little benefit. In December 1934, he was fired from his job because of frequent attacks of vertigo. By October 1934, the attacks were so severe that he refused to leave his house for fear of falling.

At least a year before his attacks of vertigo started, JB had noticed progressive hearing loss in his left ear. Along with the progressive deafness, he had a drumming noise in his left ear that seemed to vary in intensity with his deafness but not with his attacks of vertigo. His examination when he was not having vertigo was unremarkable aside from the auditory and vestibular testing. He could hear whispers 2 feet from his right ear and an ordinary speaking voice only 3 inches from the left ear. The cold caloric test showed no response on the left side after 3 minutes of irrigation, but on the right side there was normal nystagmus after 20 seconds.

The vestibular nerve section was performed by Hugh Cairns, one of the few neurosurgeons in the world at the time able to perform such a delicate procedure. Cairns was born in Port Pirie, South Australia, in 1896 (Schurr, 1990). He entered medical school at Adelaide University, but with the coming of World War I, he took leave from his medical studies. He enlisted in the Australian Army Medical Corps as a private and served in the Third Australian General Hospital at Lemnos, an island off the Dardenelles, approximately 60 miles from the Anzac beach. Following the evacuation from Gallipoli in December 1915, Cairns returned to Adelaide and completed his medical degree, receiving first-class honors. He received a Rhodes scholarship in 1916 to pursue his studies in surgical pathology at Oxford. However, he re-enrolled in the army, this time as a captain in the Medical Corps, serving in France, where he participated in the Battle of the Marne. Following the armistice and with the intercession from the Master of Balliol, he was granted an early discharge from the Medical Corps so that he could pursue his studies at Oxford. In 1921, he gained his FRCS (Fellow in the Royal College of Surgeons) and he married the youngest daughter of the Master of Balliol.

After receiving a Rockefeller Traveling Fellowship, Cairns worked with Harvey Cushing at the Peter Bent Brigham Hospital in Boston from 1926 to 1927. Cairns thrived on working long hours with little sleep. He later commented that Gallipoli and the Battle of the Mame were nothing compared to the physical stress of a year as Cushing's neurosurgical resident (Fulton, 1946). Cushing and Cairns shared not only the same initials but also the same irascible personality that often terrified their junior staff. They both believed that one worked until a job was done. There was no such thing as a specific number of hours in a workday or workweek. While operating, Cairns demanded that everything had to be highly regimented with conversation limited to only absolutely necessary details. One of his trainees, Peter Schurr (1990), recalled that

> if some hapless assistant moved too slowly, sucked too hard or too long, or misused the diathermy electrode, he would be told about it in no uncertain terms. If one's foot got in the way, it would be gently kicked, followed by the remark that a neurosurgeon should move with the quickness and lightness of a ballet dancer. (p. 190)

On the other hand, Cairns was noted for being remarkably courteous and kind to his patients and to their families. He was well aware of the life and death nature of the illnesses he dealt with and would spend long hours counseling the patient and family regarding the surgical options. Like Harvey Cushing, he was acutely aware of the importance of monitoring outcome in his patients, and he maintained careful long-term follow-up whenever possible. Whenever an outcome was unsuccessful, he nearly always obtained permission for postmortem examination because of the ties developed with the patient and the patient's family. He believed that the study of pathology was the key to understanding disease and was an invaluable tool for teaching.

At that time, it was traditional to group together all inner ear causes of vertigo under the indiscriminate label of "Ménière's syndrome." Whether there was a Ménière's disease with specific pathological features or whether there were many different diseases that resulted in the combination of symptoms described by Ménière was unknown. Some clinicians argued that one could identify a clinical syndrome with a characteristic combination of auditory and vestibular symptoms, but without a specific pathology, most remained skeptical (Hallpike and Cairns, 1938). Regardless of the cause of these inner ear symptoms, however, in the case of JB, Cairns had conclusive evidence that they originated from the left inner ear (because of the hearing loss and absent caloric response), and prior experience had convinced him that cutting the vestibular nerve could relieve the vertigo attacks (because the abnormal signals originating from the inner ear could not reach the brain). The surgery on

JB was performed on December 18, 1934. Cairns noted that the operation was unusually difficult because of the thickness and hardness of the temporal bone (Hallpike and Cairns, 1938). Because of this, the opening in the temporal bone was smaller than usual, but still he was able to cut the left vestibular nerve and part of the left cochlear nerve (see Figure 1.1). Division of the nerve went smoothly, although throughout the operation, the patient's blood pressure remained unusually high. Later that evening after the operation, "he became restless, and during the night unconscious, with rising pulse rate and temperature, stertorous and bubbly breathing, small fixed pupils, absent corneal reflexes, flaccid limbs, diminished or absent tendon and plantar reflexes, and raised blood pressure" (Hallpike and Cairns, 1938, p. 57). Cairns reopened the surgical site 12 hours after the first operation and noted prominent swelling of the left cerebellar hemisphere, associated with herniation of the cerebellar tissue through the foramen magnum. He relieved the pressure by removing part of the swollen cerebellum, after which the patient showed some improvement, although he never fully regained consciousness. The postoperative course was complicated with progressive pulmonary symptoms due to pneumonia. Despite efforts to suction and drain the purulent fluid from his lungs, JB died on December 21, 1934. An autopsy performed 6 hours after death showed that both lungs were congested and there were nodules of bronchopneumonia in the right lung. Examination of the brain showed a large hemorrhage into the left cerebellar hemisphere extending across the midline. Both inner ears and their bony capsules were cut out with a saw and placed in storage in 4% formaldehyde solution.

The temporal bones of JB sat in formaldehyde at the London Hospital for more than 1 year before Cairns became aware of Charles Hallpike's interest in temporal bone pathology. After carefully scrutinizing Hallpike in a lengthy interview, Cairns decided to entrust him with the temporal bones (Jefferson, 1959). Hallpike received the specimens at the Ferens Institute on April 22, 1936, and began the tedious process of preparing the specimens for microscopic examination (as described previously). When Hallpike was finally able to examine the histological sections under a microscope, he found a prominent distension of the entire membranous labyrinth that he called endolymphatic hydrops (Figure 13.1). The hydrops was most pronounced in the saccule and scala media of the cochlea, with obliteration of the perilymphatic spaces of the vestibule and the scala vestibuli, respectively. The organ of Corti was compressed and degenerated, but the tissue specimens showed significant postmortem artifact so that it was difficult to be certain how much of these changes was due to the hydrops and how much was due to artifact. Just as Hallpike was preparing these exciting findings for publication, Cairns provided him with a second temporal bone specimen.

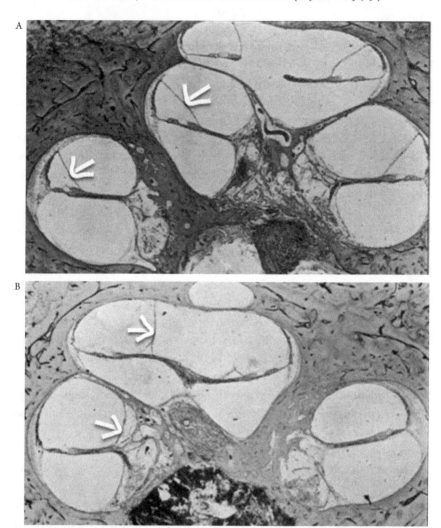

Figure 13.1 CROSS SECTIONS OF THE COCHLEA SHOWING MARKED DILATATION
OF THE COCHLEAR DUCT ON THE AFFECTED LEFT SIDE (B) COMPARED TO THE
NORMAL RIGHT SIDE (A) IN CASE 1 (JB) FROM THE 1938 REPORT BY HALLPIKE
AND CAIRNS. Arrows point to the outer membrane of the cochlear duct (Reisner's
membrane) in normal position in panel A and markedly displaced by the hydrops in
panel B. Source: From Hallpike CS, Cairns H. Observations on the pathology of Meniere's syndrome.
Proc R Soc Med 1938;31:55–74.

The second patient, JM, was a 28-year-old engineer who was referred to
Cairns for a vestibular nerve section in April 1937 because of severe recurrent attacks of vertigo dating back to 1932 (Hallpike and Cairns, 1938). JM
had noted a left-sided hearing loss, also beginning in approximately 1932, that
gradually got worse, particularly after he began having violent attacks of vertigo
in June 1936. A persistent "surging noise" in his left ear became a ringing noise

during the attacks. The healthy-looking young man could hear a watch tick at 6 inches from the left ear and 4 feet from the right. An audiogram documented a low-frequency hearing loss in the left ear, with normal hearing in the right ear. The cold caloric test produced nystagmus and moderate vertigo on both sides after irrigation with cold water for 1 minute.

A decision for surgery was made because although he was obtaining some symptomatic relief using gradually increasing doses of Luminal (a barbiturate), up to 3 grains a day, "he felt doped with the Luminal and he continued to have both mild and violent attacks, one of them in front of a prospective employer" (Hallpike and Cairns, 1938, p. 63). The operation was performed on April 22, 1937. The left vestibular nerve was sectioned in the cerebellar-pontine angle without any operative problems. In the immediate postoperative period, he had the expected spontaneous nystagmus beating to the right, and bedside hearing tests showed that his hearing in the left ear was preserved. During the second postoperative night, the patient complained of some slight headache and was restless. On the following morning, he suddenly became unconscious. He died during an emergency operation due to severe herniation of the cerebellum into the foramen magnum. Autopsy performed hours after death identified a hemorrhage into the left cerebellar hemisphere as a cause of the herniation. Hallpike and Cairns published the clinical–pathological correlation in their two patients with Ménière's syndrome in October 1938 in the *Journal of Laryngology and Otology* (Hallpike and Cairns, 1938). The gross dilatation of the endolymphatic system, particularly in the scala media of the cochlea and in the saccule, was a previously unidentified pathology. Wittmaack had used the term "hydrops labyrinthi" to describe the swelling of the membranous labyrinth due to damage from bacterial or other toxins reaching it through the round window or via the bloodstream, but the extreme uniform dilatation of the endolymphatic system was not described by Wittmaack or anyone else.

Possible Causes of Ménière's Syndrome

Regarding the mechanism for the hydrops, Hallpike and Cairns considered three possibilities: increased production of endolymph, an altered ion concentration of the endolymph, and decreased absorption of endolymph. There is a continuous circulation of endolymph thought at the time to be due to secretion in the cochlea and vestibular labyrinth and resorption in the endolymphatic sac (Figure 13.2). Hallpike and Cairns noted an obliteration of the soft connective tissue around the endolymphatic sac in the temporal bones of their patients with Ménière's syndrome and suggested that this might indicate a failure in the normal resorptive mechanism (Hallpike and Cairns, 1938). However, they found the same absence in perisaccular connective tissue in the normal temporal bone

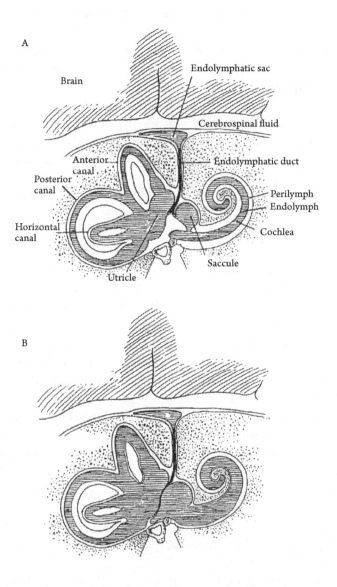

Figure 13.2 SCHEMATIC DRAWING OF THE FLUID COMPARTMENTS OF THE INNER EAR (A) AND CHANGES ASSOCIATED WITH ENDOLYMPHATIC HYDROPS (MÉNIÈRE'S DISEASE) (B). In panel B, the endolymphatic space of the cochlea and saccule are markedly dilated.

of patient JB and in 2 of 13 normal temporal bones examined. Regarding the marked dilatation in the saccule with relatively minor dilatation of the utricle, they noted that the utricular membranous wall was conspicuously more dense than the saccular wall. On average, the thickness of the utricular wall was two or three times greater than that of the saccular wall. They concluded that the saccule was simply more vulnerable to the increased endolymph pressure because of its thinner wall.

Assuming that the increased endolymph pressure and endolymphatic dilatation were the underlying pathology of Ménière's syndrome, how could this pathology explain the paroxysmal episodes of vertigo and hearing loss characteristic of the disease? For this, Hallpike and Cairns proposed a simplified model of a rigid-walled, narrow-necked vessel containing fluid and inside of it an elastic-walled balloon containing a separate fluid (Figure 13.3). The fluid inside of the balloon represented the endolymph, and the fluid in the vessel represented the perilymph. Hallpike and Cairns (1938) stated,

> A volume increase of the fluid within the balloon could clearly only lead to the ejection along the bottleneck of a corresponding amount of the surrounding fluid with little change in pressure in the system. If however the endolymph system becomes fully dilated, then a very different state of affairs is brought about. The elastic membranes are everywhere brought into contact with the rigid bony walls. . . . It is easy to see from this that the pressure change resulting from any sudden increase in volume of the fluid within the balloon would be very considerable, and would in fact be reproduced approximately by the injection into an already filled rigid vessel of an infinitesimal quantity of fluid. In other

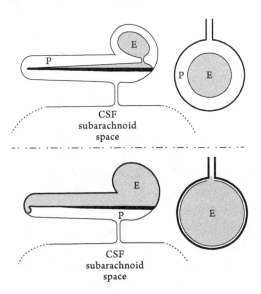

Figure 13.3 MODEL ILLUSTRATING THE MECHANISM OF ENDOLYMPHATIC HYDROPS DEVELOPED BY HALLPIKE AND CAIRNS. In the lower drawing, the endolymphatic space (E) is markedly expanded, displacing perilymph (P). CSF, cerebrospinal fluid. Source: From Hallpike CS, Cairns H. Observations on the pathology of Meniere's syndrome. *Proc R Soc Med* 1938;31:55–74.

words, once the dilatation of the endolymph system has attained its maximal degree, then the fluid system of the membranous labyrinth, from being insensitive, becomes at once extremely sensitive in its pressure response to a given volume increase of the endolymph. (p. 69)

The mechanism of the hearing loss and tinnitus with Ménière's syndrome was even more obscure than the mechanism of the episodic vertigo. Hallpike and Cairns argued that the marked increase in endolymphatic pressure could lead to a stretching of the basilar membrane within the cochlea that in turn would lead to distortion of sounds but not the hearing loss. This most likely resulted from chronic degeneration of the organ of Corti secondary to the increased pressure. Regarding the tinnitus, they noted the puzzling fact that following sectioning of the entire eighth nerve, the tinnitus continued in many patients with Ménière's syndrome. If the tinnitus resulted from degenerative changes in the organ of Corti, then it should disappear when the eighth nerve was sectioned. Hallpike and Cairns (1938) concluded, "It is only possible to attribute this [the continuation of tinnitus after eighth nerve section] to the development of certain obscure changes in the central cochlear neurons, similar in nature to those which may be responsible for painful phantom limb and other sensations of central origin" (p. 73). Interestingly, studies using functional magnetic resonance imaging have found increased activity within cortical neurons in the temporal lobe in patients with chronic tinnitus, reviving the analogy to a phantom limb syndrome (Lockwood et al., 1998).

Yamakawa Also Describes the Pathology of Ménière's Syndrome

Hallpike and Cairns began their famous 1938 article on the pathology of Ménière's syndrome as follows: "It is the purpose of this paper to describe-it is believed for the first time the pathological changes in the temporal bones of two cases of Ménière's syndrome" (p. 55). Their article was published on October 10, 1938, but unknown to the authors, a Japanese otolaryngologist, Kyoshiro Yamakawa, reported on "the pathologic changes in a Ménière's patient" at a medical congress in Kyoto, Japan, in April 1938, which was then published in a short article in German later that year. Yamakawa had also studied with Wittmaack in Germany; he was professor of otorhinolaryngology at Osaka University from 1931 to 1956 (Stahle, 1989).

Yamakawa's patient was a 61-year-old professor of gynecology at Osaka University with a 2-year history of typical Ménière's syndrome before dying suddenly of pneumonia. This patient had multiple episodes of vertigo, left-sided tinnitus, and hearing loss, with fluctuations in hearing levels and a tendency to improve between attacks. Like Hallpike and Cairns, Yamakawa found a prominent endolymphatic hydrops with marked dilatation of the cochlea and the saccule. However, Yamakawa reported that the endolymphatic duct and sac were narrow and filled with a thick colloid material, whereas Hallpike and Cairns described a normal-sized endolymphatic sac but the absence of connective tissue around the sac. Furthermore, Yamakawa found that the sensory epithelium of the cochlea and vestibular labyrinth were normal, whereas Hallpike and Cairns observed degeneration of the sensory epithelium of the organ of Corti in both cases and of the macules and cristae in their case 2. These differences might be explained on the basis of different disease durations and different degrees of postmortem artifact in the different specimens, but there is still controversy regarding whether or not damage to the sensory epithelium is a primary feature of Ménière's syndrome. Today, in our modern computerized age, the fact that investigators in Japan and England were unaware of each other's work seems inexplicable. However, one must keep in mind that in the 1930s, communication was slow, and there was an almost complete interruption of international exchanges in the lead-up to World War II.

References

Curtis JH. Employment of creosote in deafness. *Lancet* 1838a;31:328–330.

Curtis JH. Letter from Mr. J. H. Curtis. *Lancet* 1838b;31:534–535.

Eckert-Möbius A. Karl Wittmaack zum Gedächtnis. *Arch Klin Exp Ohr-Nas-u Kehlk-Heilk* 1972;210:270–273.

Fulton JF. *Harvey Cushing. A Biography.* Springfield, IL: Charles C. Thomas, 1946.

Hallpike CS, Cairns H. Observations on the pathology of Meniere's syndrome. *Proc R Soc Med* 1938;31:55-74.

Jefferson G. Memories of Hugh Cairns. *J Neurol Neurosurg Psychiatr* 1959;22:155–165.

Lockwood AH, Salvi RJ, Coad BA, et al. The functional neuroanatomy of tinnitus: Evidence for limbic system links and neural plasticity. *Neurology* 1998;50:114–120.

Pirsig W, Ulrich R. Karl Wittmaack: His life, temporal bone collection, and publications. On the 100th anniversary of his birth. *Arch Oto-Rhino-Laryngol* 1977;217:247–262.

Schurr PH. The Cairns tradition. *J Neurol Neurosurg Psychiatr* 1990;53:188–193.

Stahle J. Endolymphatic hydrops—Fiftieth anniversary. *Acta Otolaryngol (Stockh)* 1989;Suppl 468:11–16.

Stevenson RS, Guthrie D. *A History of Oto-laryngology.* Baltimore, MD: Williams & Wilkins, 1949, pp. 62–63.

Toynbee J. Effects of difficiency of cerumen on the function of hearing. *Lancet* 1838;31:422.

Toynbee J. Causes of deafness—Aural surgery. *Lancet* 1839;31:733–734.

Toynbee J. *The Diseases of the Ear: Their Nature, Diagnosis and Treatment.* London: Churchill, 1860.

Weir N. *Otolaryngology: An Illustrated History.* London: Butterworth, 1990, pp. 74–77.

Whitteridge D, Merton PA. Charles Skinner Hallpike, 19 July1900–26 September 1979. *Biographical Memoirs of Fellows of the Royal Society* 1984;30:283–294.

Yamakawa K. Über die pathologische Veränderung bei einem Meniere-Kranken. *Z Oto-Rhino-Laryngol Organ Japan ORL Gesellschaft* 1938;44:192–193.

14

Hallpike's Formative Years

The Indian Connection

Charles Skinner Hallpike was born on July 19, 1900, in Muree, a small hill station and health resort in the northernmost area of what was then India (Whitteridge and Merton, 1984) and now a part of Pakistan, just northeast of the capitol of Islamabad. He was baptized at the Church of St. James, in Delhi, India, on December 25, 1900. This was one of the three places of worship—a Hindu temple, a mosque, and a Christian church—built by Hallpike's great-grandfather, James Skinner (1778–1841), a colorful soldier of fortune of the Internecine and Imperial Wars that were part of the British domination of India at the turn of the 19th century (Mason, 1979). James Skinner's father, Hercules Skinner, was a Scot and a captain in the East India Company who married a Rajput, a member of the Hindu caste of noble descent. James's mother supposedly committed suicide when her daughters (Skinner's sisters) were taken away from her to be taught to read and write and behave like English ladies. Skinner's father knew that no Rajput would marry their mixed-race daughters and no Englishman would marry them unless they could read and write. James Skinner wanted to be a soldier like his father, but he could not be commissioned because his mother was an Indian. He was as brown as his mother, and Hindi was his first language. Despite being apprenticed to a local printer, James engineered an introduction to General de Boigne, and he was commissioned as an ensign in de Boigne's private army, serving the Maharaja Scindia. James Skinner was a very successful soldier and a natural diplomat. At its height, his regiment was a brigade of three cavalry regiments known as "Skinner's Horse." Such was its reputation and that of its founder that the name has perpetuated down to today's Indian Army. He was awarded the Order of the Bath (C.B.), but first he had to be commissioned in His Majesty's Forces. He was commissioned as a lieutenant colonel and then received his C.B. at the same ceremony.

While lying wounded on a battlefield in 1800, James Skinner was said to have sworn an oath: "I will build a church for the worship of my father's God and a temple for my mother's gods and a mosque for the God of those who follow Mohammed and have fought by my side." Skinner believed that one should commit to a faith and that the commitment was more important to God than what faith was chosen (Mason, 1979). Skinner died in 1841 at the age of 64. He was initially buried at Hansi and after a period of 40 days was disentered and brought to Delhi escorted by 200 men of Skinner's Horse. He was ultimately buried in a vault of white marble in the church of his father's god, Skinner's church, the church where his great-grandson, Charles Skinner Hallpike, was later baptized (Figure 14.1).

Rosamund Helen Skinner, the granddaughter of James Skinner, married Frank Hallpike, a jeweler from west London, in February 1898. Soon after their marriage, they moved to India, where Charles Skinner Hallpike was born. While in India, Frank Hallpike's occupation was listed as "landed proprietor." The Hallpikes moved back to London when Charles was 3 years old. They lived in a Victorian terraced house in Hammersmith, a predominantly working-class western suburban neighborhood. Charles's mother Rosamund was proud of her Indian heritage, artifacts of which she proudly displayed throughout her home in Hammersmith. On entering the drawing room, on the first floor, it was like moving straight from Hammersmith to India. There were tiger skins, artwork from India, and picture books of exotic animals. Rosamund was a quiet, dignified lady, very Indian in her appearance. Frank Hallpike apparently was not very successful as a jeweler and was very much in the background in family activities.

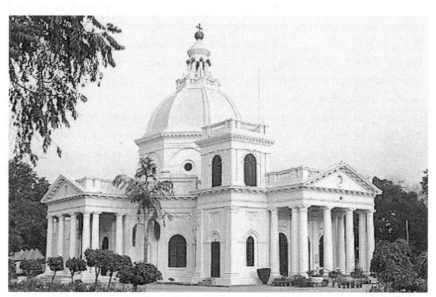

Figure 14.1 SKINNER'S CHURCH (ST. JAMES CHURCH), THE OLDEST CHURCH IN DELHI, INDIA. It has three porches and a central octagonal dome.

Early Education and Dealing with Legg–Perthes Disease

Charles was an excellent young athlete, being particularly fond of soccer. His life was turned upside down, however, when at age 12 he suffered what seemed to be a minor injury in a soccer match at school (Baloh, 2000). The pain in his hip initially was of little concern; his main concern was to get back into the game. When the pain persisted, he underwent a series of examinations and finally was diagnosed with Legg–Perthes disease. The cause of Legg–Perthes disease is unknown, but it results in a temporary cutoff of blood supply to the head of the femoral bone that fits into the hip socket. What follows is a vicious cycle of small areas of bone necrosis followed by attempts at repair with new bone growth. The abnormal growth affects the developing femoral head and how well it fits into the hip socket, resulting in severe pain when walking. Because of the condition, young Hallpike spent long periods of his childhood propped up in bed with weights hanging from his feet. Charles's school friends would take turns visiting to entertain him during his many months spent on his back. He had a half-sized billiard table set up in his room, and he learned to play billiards from his bed. The table was not level and the cushions gave uneven bounces, but he learned all of its idiosyncrasies and soon became an expert player. Story has it that an amateur billiard champion who lived in the area was invited in for a game and was soundly defeated (son Jeremy Hallpike, personal communication, 1998).

Despite his medical problems, Charles was an excellent student and became a classical scholar at St. Paul's School, graduating in 1919. His older sister Muriel had gone with him to view the results of his matriculation and said he could not have passed because his name was not there. He said, "Of course it's not there you silly girl, it's on the Honours Board" (Jeremy Hallpike, personal communication, 1998).

Medical Training

He began his medical training at Guy's Hospital with a scholarship in the arts in 1919 (Whitteridge and Merton, 1984). His most influential teacher was the physiologist Pembrey, who taught him the importance of understanding the pathophysiology of disease processes. He received the Beaney Prize in pathology and obtained his medical degree in 1924. At that time, Guy's Hospital was known for its practical clinical approach, with little interest in academic endeavors. Despite his limited basic training, however, Hallpike had a good foundation in physics and physiology that would later be the key for his academic achievements.

After graduating from medical school, he was appointed House Surgeon to T. B. Layton in the Ear, Nose and Throat Department at Guy's Hospital. He took his Membership of the Royal College of Physicians of London and followed with his Fellowship of the Royal College of Surgeons. Hallpike gained surgical experience at Cheltenham General Hospital. In 1929, he became the Berhard Baron research fellow at the Ferens Institute of Otology at the Middlesex Hospital in London, and he published his first scientific paper the following year. His early publications were mostly of work on the physiology of hearing and the scientific basis of hearing tests. He was awarded the Gamble Prize for Otological Research in 1934, an award he would receive again in 1947. Physiology, however, was not enough. He was convinced of the importance of the study of pathology for understanding disease processes. Hallpike believed that to be effective, the clinical scientist needed to have a number of techniques available to him. He was at the forefront of understanding the importance of the multidisciplinary approach to the elucidation of clinical problems.

Personal Life

In July 1935, Charles Hallpike married Barbara Lee Anderson, daughter of a local brewer Charles Anderson. They had three children—two sons and a daughter. Unlike his parents' home, there was nothing Indian in Charles Hallpike's home. Charles's complexion was naturally dark, unusual for an Englishman, and became even darker in the sun. Although he was sensitive about the perceived social stigma associated with his mixed-race Indian ancestry, he did not readily acknowledge this. However, it would come to the surface when he would tell funny stories about one or the other of his uncles who continued to live in India and who visited occasionally (Jeremy Hallpike, personal communication, 1998).

Hallpike had a reputation of being rather unapproachable. On the other hand, he was comfortable with his clinical peers, and he had a protective attitude to the people who worked for him. He was innately loyal and courteous. Hallpike tended to eschew small talk at work as well as socially (Jeremy Hallpike, personal communication, 1998). Perhaps a reflection of his surgical background, he was interested in exchanging facts rather than ideas—certainly poorly sorted out ideas or, as he would say, "lucubrations." Abstract intellectual conversation held little appeal for him. However, he had a quick wit and a black sense of humor. On one occasion, while he was sitting in his laboratory sectioning the temporal bone specimen of a former patient, he received a note that a man of the same name as his former patient had called to see him. "Good God," he said, "the man's come back for his ears" (Stahle, 1989).

His entry into a conversation often took the form of an apparently innocent question but one to which there was only one correct answer. For example, he might say to a ranking cleric in full flight of the meaning of Christianity, "What I've always wanted to know is what exactly was it that the Protestants protested about?" The correct answer, that they protested against the Edict of Worms of 1529 to put down the Reformation, could not be provided by the "expert," who would lose the ascendancy. When the word "parameter" suddenly became a buzzword and was being used to explain something to him, he would say, "I do wish you would explain this word to me." Explanations would always be woolly and in terms of some sort of dependent variable, whereas a parameter is an independent constant (e.g., Mach's number). It was a Socratic approach, part of his technique for penetrating what he suspected to be a knowledgeable veneer.

Hallpike's daughter-in-law Jane recalled how he tended to exaggerate and make things up with a completely dead-pan face. When they first met, he quickly put her to the test with a horrifying story about how one of his wife's mother's five husbands blew his brains out over the dining room ceiling with his service revolver. She managed to laugh and thereby passed his test. When someone asked him if he was still in *Who's Who*, he replied at once, "No, I'm now in What's What" (daughter in-law Jane Hallpike, personal communication, 1998). The constant hip pain from Legg–Perthes disease finally became unbearable, and in his late 50s, Hallpike underwent a Girdlestone's operation to produce a pseudoarthrosis. After this, he was able to sit comfortably but could not walk for any distance. He referred to the few steps that he could take as the "Girdlestone's gavotte."

Hallpike the Inventor

Hallpike was an ingenious designer of equipment even though he had no formal engineering background (Baloh, 2000). One of his proudest achievements was the development of a monocular microscope for examining the ear. Although the microscope never became popular with other otologists, to Hallpike's amusement, poultry farmers adopted it for sexing day-old chicks. He designed magnifying spectacles that were widely sold. Even his dentist bought a pair. A Hallpike Operating Headlamp was also manufactured and marketed by the same company. As was customary at the time, the Medical Research Council that employed him held the patents on these inventions and the Council received the royalties. The company promised Hallpike free glasses for life, although in later years that arrangement was renounced on the grounds of "previous administration and nothing documented" (Jeremy Hallpike, personal communication, 1998).

Appointment at Queen Square

At the end of an association of almost 10 years with the Ferens Institute, supported by a succession of short-term research fellowships, Hallpike found himself entering 1939 without a firm position and with uncertain prospects. World War II was beginning, but he was unable to enlist because of his chronic hip problem. Three men with markedly different backgrounds came to Hallpike's rescue and provided the turning point in his career. Sir Edward Mellanby was a dynamic and highly influential secretary of the British Medical Research Council (MRC) that strongly encouraged research that had an immediate bearing on human health (Dale, 1955). Mellanby had set up a series of MRC units, each of which emphasized a different subspecialty.

The second person to have an effect on Hallpike's career was E. A. Carmichael, director of the MRC Neurological Research Unit at Queen Square, a unit that was noted for its multidisciplinary approach to understanding the mechanism of neurologic diseases. Mellanby was aware of Hallpike's work, particularly the work on the pathology of Ménière's disease, and he suggested to Carmichael that Hallpike would be a good addition to the MRC at Queen Square.

The third key player was Terence Cawthorne, the senior ear, nose, and throat (ENT) surgeon at Queen Square. Mellanby and Carmichael convinced Cawthorne to offer Hallpike a clinical appointment in the hospital; thus, in early 1940, at the age of 39, Hallpike was appointed to the established scientific staff of the MRC and to the honorary consultant staff of the ENT department at Queen Square. Hallpike's new position was highly unconventional in those days, namely a research appointment with the privileges and status of a clinical consultant. A few years later, in 1944, his clinical appointment was institutionalized through the new position of Aural Physician at Queen Square. His position was further consolidated through the establishment in 1944 of the Otological Research Unit of the MRC and his appointment as its director. He held both of these appointments until the time of his retirement in 1965.

Hallpike's Colleagues at Queen Square

When Hallpike arrived at Queen Square in 1940, his first priority was to establish a temporal bone laboratory. He was fortunate to find two young technicians, Best in histology and Bolum a mechanic, who stayed with him throughout his career. Between the three of them, technical requirements were met through improvisation, and the laboratories were filled with ingenious homemade devices. In addition to his skills in preparing histological slides, Best had a knack with photography and became an expert at the specialized "macrophotography" used for temporal bone studies. In collaboration with researchers at the National Physical Laboratory and the National Institute for Medical Research, Best, Hallpike, and colleagues developed a new microtomy knife made of stainless steel with a Stellite edge (Best et al., 1956). This cobalt–chromium–tungsten–carbon alloy, which was sharpened on a special machine after every few cuts, allowed them to produce ultrathin sections of the hard temporal bone specimens for the first time. Bolum helped to build the rotational chair and other electromechanical devices that were being brought into use in the new Otoneurology Laboratory.

Although Cawthorne was initially supportive of Hallpike's appointment, it was not long before a degree of rivalry developed between the two men (Jeremy Hallpike, personal communication, 1998). The key issue seemed to be one of ascendancy. Cawthorne was a highly distinguished ENT surgeon who had led the way with otosclerosis surgery in London. He would hold the presidency of the Royal Society of Medicine and was ultimately knighted for his wide services to medicine and otology. Perhaps he believed that Hallpike owed a loyalty to him for his support in his original appointment that would otherwise have gone to a surgeon of his choosing in private practice. It should be borne in mind that in those days, before the National Health Service was introduced in 1946, almost all consultant appointments were under the honorary system—that is, unpaid. At the beginning, there were ambiguities about Hallpike's appointment that encouraged a belief that his research was somehow under Cawthorne's auspices with authorship implications and the right to use of material for lecture purposes. Hallpike would have none of this. The authority for publication of the work carried out under Hallpike's direction was his alone. These differences were settled administratively, up to a point, when in 1944 Hallpike was appointed to the new position of Aural Physician at Queen Square. At the same time, he was made director of the newly created Otological Research Unit. Nevertheless, rivalry between the two men continued throughout their stay at Queen Square.

War Years

Just before World War II, the Hallpike family moved to a house on The Ridgeway in Mill Hill across from the United Kingdom Optical Works, a factory built by Bausch and Lomb a few years earlier. During the war, a short distance from the factory was the Inglis barracks of the Middlesex regiment, and just down from that was a huge depot for all sorts of wheeled vehicles, including tanks. Going in the other direction along The Ridgeway was the headquarters of the Women's Royal Naval Service and a large ammunition dump with an array of camouflaged bunkers. Fortunately for the Hallpikes, German bombing of the area, although heavy during the early part of the war, was almost entirely at night and poorly directed.

Throughout the war, the windows in their house were sealed over for anti-splintering protection so they could not see out. On a daily basis, one heard the intermittent sounds of the warning sirens and the continuous sound of the all-clear. Even the slightest show of light brought a warning knock from the air raid precautions warden. Initially, the family went to a nearby air raid shelter or hid in a storage area under the stairs, but they later just stayed in the bedrooms and took potluck. Their oldest son Jeremy recalled the noise of the planes, the anti-aircraft fire from all around, and above all the whine of the falling bombs. He collected the pieces of anti-aircraft shrapnel from the garden each morning and marched up and down alongside the soldiers as they moved to and from their barracks. They lived from day-to-day according to their ration books—so many points for this and so many points for that.

The MRC was the government organization responsible for finding official answers to biomedical questions. During the war, Hallpike served on the Military Personnel Research Committee of the MRC. He also served on the Flying Personnel Research Committee of the Air Ministry. One of the first crises that he had to deal with was deafness in tank crews after they fired the main guns. This was causing great concern with the Matilda tanks that were being supplied to the British forces in North Africa in 1940. Hallpike (as quoted by Jeremy Hallpike, personal communication, 1998) recalled how he visited the boardroom of the large automotive company involved in the manufacture of Matilda tanks to gather relevant information:

> All I'd taken with me was a child's exercise book. I interrogated the chairman and other members present for a full morning and wrote it all down. Then I went away. I think the Board were very taken aback by this approach.

Hallpike's solution was a more efficient ear plug, which was made available within a few weeks.

Later during the war, he worked on the development of lightweight body armor to reduce the mortality from shrapnel and metal fragment injuries. Because soldiers disliked carrying additional weight and having their movements restricted, much effort went into alloy selection and design in terms of optimum arrangement of the webbing-linked panels. Hallpike became personally involved in the practical field testing of the new lightweight body armor, an experience that he said made him appreciative of the quality of the German ammunition. Looking back, he would sometimes state how fortunate Britain was to have survived the war with Germany. His work on these high-level wartime committees brought him into contact with many of the leading scientists of the day.

Each day, Hallpike rode the 240 bus down the hill to Mill Hill East station on the northern line of the underground (subway). He had to change at Leicester Square to the Piccadilly line, and there were three stops until Russell Square, next door to the National Hospital at Queen Square. The journey was 45 minutes door-to-door. The Hallpike family purchased its first automobile in 1948, a green Rover 75. Because of his Legg–Perthes disease, Hallpike and his technician Bolum worked out a hand clutch, a special seat, and a gear lever that extended upward to suit him. Much time was spent keeping the car immaculate. Jeremy recalled that the hood became quite worn away with the frequent polishing.

Queen Square Neurotology Clinic

As director of an otologic unit in an institution with such a rich tradition in neurology, Hallpike entered into competition with his illustrious neurological colleagues at Queen's Square. He had no desire for membership in the "baggy trousers brigade," a term used by Roger Gilliatt for down at heel scientists and provincial doctors. He acquired beautifully tailored suits from Henry Poole in Saville Row that also served to disguise the deformity of his hip. His hair was always cut by Mr. Green at Penhaligon's on Jermyn Street. Perhaps only Macdonald Critchley, famous neurologist and dean of the Institute at Queen Square, could rival him in appearance and manner in the all-important Front Hall of the hospital. Hallpike never failed to acknowledge his sense of genuine privilege at every opportunity to examine and report on the patients who were referred to him by his neurological colleagues. They soon found that his careful otoneurological examinations were very useful in the clinical management of their patients. The D Room NeuroOtology Clinic was the public face of the Otological Research Unit. He was able to obtain the firm support and friendship of Wylie McKissock, who dominated neurosurgery in the London area at that time: "Woe betide any resident who allowed a patient with an eighth nerve tumor to come to surgery without having had his Hallpikery!" (Jeremy Hallpike, personal communication, 1998). Later, when Hallpike was elected a Fellow of the Royal Society in 1956, the first otologist ever accorded that honor, it was Critchley, the then-senior neurologist at Queen Square, who was reported to have said, "Well, Charles, we will have to take you seriously now." With Carmichael's retirement and Roger Gilliatt's appointment as the first Professor of Neurology, Hallpike's MRC Otology unit was under increasing scrutiny once more. Some of the senior neurologists were alarmed about the enlargement of these "scientific empires" as they saw the ongoing developments in Hallpike's unit. Sir Charles Symonds is reported to have said, "You are like a cancer, Hallpike, metastasizing and then devouring the host" (Jeremy Hallpike, personal communication, 1998).

Hallpike began his career in neurotology by thoroughly reading the works of Bárány. He was well grounded in the German literature and frequently quoted Bárány in his publications. Interestingly, there were remarkable parallels in the careers of Hallpike and Bárány. Both experienced physical disabilities in childhood that limited their physical activity throughout life and no doubt had a major contribution to their generally perceived aloof personalities. Both had dramatic early successes that propelled their academic career— Bárány with the caloric test and Hallpike with the pathology of Ménière's disease. They were clinicians first and researchers second, and much of their work was directed toward developing reliable clinical diagnostic tests. Each had a stubborn streak in his personality that allowed him to stick with research projects until they were completed but at the same time prevented him from accepting new and sometimes better explanations for his research findings. Finally, both had a fascination with the central nervous system, even though they trained as otologic surgeons and had little background in neuroanatomy or neurophysiology. Their willingness to address neurologic disorders and neurologic causes of otologic symptoms (other otologists tended to ignore them) redefined the subspecialty of neurotology.

References

Baloh RW. Charles Skinner Hallpike and the beginnings of neurotology. *Neurology* 2000;54: 2138–2146.

Best C, Fordham S, Hallpike CS, et al. Notes on the technique of temporal bone microtomy. *Br Med Bull* 1956;12:93–100.

Dale HH. Edward Mellanby. *Biographical Memoirs of Fellows of the Royal Society* 1955;1:193–222.

Mason P. *Skinner of Skinner's Horse: A Fictional Portrait.* London: Andre Deutsch, 1979.

Stahle J. Endolymphatic hydrops—Fiftieth anniversary. *Acta Otolaryngol (Stockh)* 1989;Suppl 468:11–16.

Whitteridge D, Merton PA. Charles Skinner Hallpike, 19 July1900–26 September 1979. *Biographical Memoirs of Fellows of the Royal Society* 1984;30:283–294.

15

Hallpike's Caloric Test

Since Bárány introduced the caloric test in the clinic, various attempts were made to improve the sensitivity and reliability, although there was no generally accepted method for performing the test. Kobrak (1918) repeatedly infused 5 cc of water of increasing coldness until he arrived at a threshold value for nystagmus production, but this was a tedious process that was not very sensitive and certainly not practical. Hallpike concluded that greater precision could be obtained by measuring the duration of induced nystagmus because it was the attribute that he could most reliably measure (Fitzgerald and Hallpike, 1942). Regarding the question of which temperature of water and how long to infuse the water, Hallpike chose water at 30° and 44°C (7°C below and above body temperature) and allowed it to flow for 40 seconds. These temperatures were generally well tolerated, and the comparatively large quantity of water and rapid flow minimized errors due to misdirecting the stream within the ear canal.

Preparing the Water

Hallpike developed an elaborate method for preparing the caloric temperature baths. A 2-pint metal can was filled with hot or cold water directly out of the tap, and by using a thermometer mounted on a perforated wooden plunger, the water in the can was mixed until it was 1°C above the temperature required. The final adjustment was then made by running cold water around the base of the container while constantly mixing the water within. The can was then hung on a stand, and the water was delivered to the ear through a rubber tube whose 4-mm diameter tip directed the stream into the ear canal. Approximately 8 ounces of water was delivered into the canal over 40 seconds. Water in the feed tube was always run off before starting the irrigation, and the stream of water was directed toward the posterior wall of the ear canal.

For the test, the patient would lie on a couch with head raised approximately 30 degrees above the horizontal so that the horizontal semicircular canal was in the vertical plane (Figure 15.1). The patient was asked to fixate on a mark on the ceiling. The duration of the induced nystagmus after each of the four caloric stimuli was measured by two observers stationed on each side of the couch using light reflected from the head mirrors from a source above and behind the patient's head. Hallpike chose to measure the time from the beginning of the stimulation to the end of the nystagmus response using a stopwatch.

He chose not to measure the duration from the onset of nystagmus because he argued that this was often difficult to accurately identify and although there may be some difference in the rate of transmission of the thermal wave through the bone to the labyrinth in different individuals, it was not likely that there would be variations in this transmission time between the two ears in any given individual. It took approximately 4 minutes for each single caloric test, and 5 minutes was allowed between each test so that additive effects would be avoided. Thus, the standard bithermal caloric test took at least 30 minutes to perform (not including the preparation time).

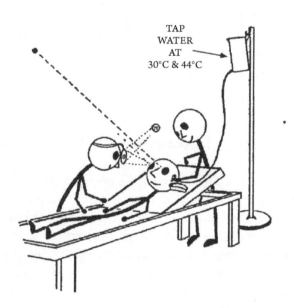

TAP
WATER
AT
30°C & 44°C

Figure 15.1 SCHEMATIC ILLUSTRATION OF HALLPIKE'S BITHERMAL CALORIC TEST. Source: From Fitzgerald G, Hallpike CS. Studies in human vestibular function: 1. Observations on the directional preponderance ("Nystagmusbereitschaft") of caloric nystagmus resulting from cerebral lesions. *Brain* 1942;65:115–137.

Hallpike's Caloric Chart

A simple chart was used to summarize the results of the bithermal caloric test (Figure 15.2). The chart consisted of two continuous lines, each representing a total of a 3-minute period, subdivided into 10-second intervals. The duration of nystagmus after the two 30°C stimuli was marked above and below the upper line and the duration after the two 44°C stimuli on the lower line. Two characteristic abnormal patterns were identified. With a canal paresis, the duration of nystagmus to both cool and warm water on one side was decreased compared to that on the opposite side. With a directional preponderance, nystagmus in one direction was stronger than nystagmus in the opposite direction, regardless of which ear was stimulated with hot or cold water.

Hallpike routinely performed his bithermal caloric tests on all patients he saw in his Queen Square Otology Clinic. A young associate, under his watchful eye, typically prepared the water baths. Hallpike could be very testy if a problem

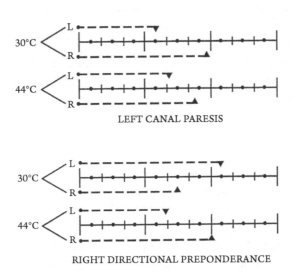

Figure 15.2 Charts developed by Hallpike to summarize the results of his standard caloric test. With a canal paresis, the duration of nystagmus after left 30°C and left 44°C water is deceased compared to the duration of nystagmus after stimulation of the opposite ear. With a directional preponderance, the duration of nystagmus after right 30°C and left 44°C water is decreased compared with stimulation with left 30°C and right 44°C water. Source: From Fitzgerald G, Hallpike CS. Studies in human vestibular function: 1. Observations on the directional preponderance ("Nystagmusbereitschaft") of caloric nystagmus resulting from cerebral lesions. *Brain* 1942;65:115–137.

arose, so his young associates often dreaded this part of their duties. In later years, as Hallpike developed an international reputation, visiting specialists, many from America, flooded his department. To deal with this onslaught of visitors, Hallpike devised a screening procedure administered by his secretary. The visitor was given a sample case history and a chart with the results of the caloric test. Hallpike only received those who could properly interpret the caloric test and make a correct diagnosis (Stahle, 1989).

The Meaning of a Directional Preponderance

When he arrived at Queen Square, Hallpike was fascinated by the work of Bauer and Leidler at the University of Vienna, who in 1912 reported that removing a cerebral hemisphere in the rabbit caused an asymmetry of post-rotational nystagmus. After the operation, when rotation toward the intact hemisphere was suddenly stopped, the post-rotational nystagmus was much brisker than after stopping rotation toward the damaged hemisphere. Based on Ewald's second law, which states that when an animal is rotated to the right at a constant velocity and then suddenly stopped, the post-rotational nystagmus is primarily due to excitation of the left inner ear, Bauer and Leidler concluded that each cerebral hemisphere gives rise to an increased sensitivity of the inner ear on that side. Thus, if you remove one cerebral hemisphere, you create an imbalance between the inner ears, with the contralateral (opposite) inner ear being more sensitive because of its intact cerebral hemisphere. In 1923, Dusser de Barenne and de Kleyn confirmed the experiments of Bauer and Leidler, but in addition to evaluating post-rotational nystagmus, they studied caloric-induced nystagmus. Because the caloric stimulus allowed them to activate each inner ear independently with hot and cold water, they found that removing a cerebral hemisphere did not facilitate the response of one inner ear but, rather, facilitated nystagmus in one direction compared to the opposite direction. For example, they found that removing the right cerebral hemisphere resulted in stronger nystagmus when either the left ear was irrigated with cold water or the right ear was irrigated with warm water (a so-called right directional preponderance). Dusser de Barenne and de Kleyn suggested that this directional preponderance of caloric-induced nystagmus might be useful in the diagnosis of cerebral lesions. It must be remembered that at that time, there were no good ways to image the brain.

Hallpike conducted a series of experiments studying the phenomenon of directional preponderance with a young research fellow working in his laboratory, Gerald Fitzgerald. In a paper published in the journal *Brain* in 1942, Fitzgerald and Hallpike reported on the results of caloric testing in 20 patients with focal brain lesions using the new standardized caloric test. The location of the lesion was established either on clinical grounds alone or by direct evidence of operative or postmortem findings. In the 10 cases in which the lesions involved the temporal lobes, there was a directional preponderance of caloric nystagmus toward the side of the lesion, whereas in the other 10 cases with lesions that did not involve the temporal lobes, none had a directional preponderance of caloric nystagmus. As did Dusser de Barenne and de Kleyn (1923), they suggested that identification of a directional preponderance on caloric testing might prove useful for localizing brain lesions. The posterior temporal lobes presumably exert a balanced tonic effect on the vestibular nuclei so that a lesion on one side results in an imbalance of this tonic effect producing a directional preponderance on caloric testing.

Hallpike and colleagues also observed a directional preponderance on caloric testing after lesions of the inner ear and vestibular nerve (Cawthorne et al., 1942). Not surprisingly, if one destroys an inner ear on one side, the resulting spontaneous nystagmus produces a strong directional preponderance toward the intact side. The spontaneous nystagmus adds to the caloric-induced nystagmus in the same direction and subtracts from that in the opposite direction. This spontaneous nystagmus typically disappears within several days to a week. However, they observed a directional preponderance toward the intact side even after the spontaneous nystagmus disappeared. This persistent directional preponderance presumably resulted from unbalanced tonus emanating from the unaffected inner ear.

Importance of Tonic Signals Originating from the Inner Ears

In the early 1920s, Magnus clearly showed the importance of inner ear tone on the eye and body musculature when he destroyed a single inner ear in the rabbit. Immediately after the inner ear was removed, the head and body were twisted (Grunddrehung) toward the side of the surgery (Magnus, 1924). This extreme posture was due to a decrease in tone of extensor muscles on the side of the damaged ear and an increased tone of extensor muscles on the unaffected side. There was a spontaneous nystagmus with the rapid phase toward the unaffected side but also a tonic deviation of the eyes toward the side of the surgery. Magnus attributed these effects on postural and ocular muscles to an imbalance in spontaneous tonus originating from the remaining intact inner ear.

The first clue as to the nature of the inner ear tonus came when an American biologist at Clark University, Hudson Hoagland, recorded spontaneous firing in the nerve from the lateral line organ of the catfish, the primitive forerunner of the inner ear (Hoagland, 1933). In 1936, Otto Löwenstein and Alexander

Sand, working at the University of Birmingham, England, recorded spontaneous activity originating from the nerve supplying the horizontal semicircular canal in the dogfish. These investigators went on to show that resting action potential discharge in the horizontal canal nerve increased with endolymph flow toward the ampulla and decreased with endolymph flow away from the ampulla. Thus, they provided an explanation for Breuer's observation that a single semicircular canal could sense movement of endolymph in both directions. As noted previously, endolymph flow toward or away from the ampulla increased or decreased the spontaneous tonic activity in the afferent nerve.

In 1958, Ledoux showed that there were spontaneous action potentials originating from all of the nerve branches of the sensory receptors of the frog inner ear, just as Löwenstein and Sand had seen in the horizontal canal nerve of the dogfish. Over subsequent years, many investigators studying several different mammals including primates showed that this is a universal phenomenon—that is, spontaneous action potentials originate from all of the sensory receptors of the inner ear.

Controversy Regarding the Effect of Cortical Lesions

In 1959, a controversy arose regarding the effect of cortical lesions on vestibular nystagmus when investigators in Germany reported that the directional preponderance to caloric-induced nystagmus that occurred in patients with lesions of the posterior temporal lobe was directed to the side opposite the lesion, not toward the side of the lesion as reported by Fitzgerald and Hallpike in 1942 (Hakas and Kornhuber, 1959). They electrically recorded the nystagmus (electronystagmography) with eyes closed rather than with visual fixation as done by Hallpike (Figure 15.3). To prove that this was the explanation for the difference in findings between the two groups, Hallpike and associates at Queen Square conducted another series of experiments with caloric testing in patients with lesions of the posterior temporal lobe using their traditional caloric test with visual fixation and then repeating the test with electrical eye movement recordings with the eyes closed. They were able to show that in many cases the directional preponderance of caloric nystagmus changed directions with eyes closed (Carmichael et al., 1961).

Hallpike believed that this was a good example of the danger of recording vestibular caloric-induced nystagmus with eyes closed and argued that the test should be performed with visual fixation as his group had originally proposed. There was merit to both sides of the argument about directional preponderance and temporal lobe lesions, but probably the most important outcome of

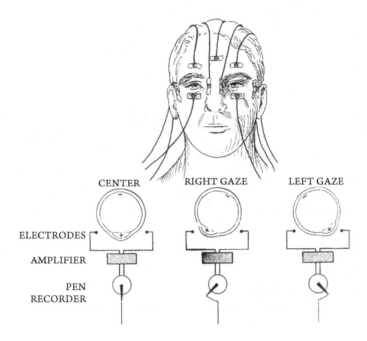

Figure 15.3 ELECTRONYSTAGMOGRAPHY. The difference in electrical potential between the cornea and the retina acts as an electrical dipole, oriented in the direction of the long axis of the eyeball. In relation to a remote electrode (in this case on the forehead), an electrode placed next to the eye becomes more positive when the eye rotates toward it and less positive when the eye rotates in the opposite direction. Recordings are usually made with a three-electrode system using differential amplification. Source: From Baloh RW, Honrubia V. *Clinical Neurophysiology of the Vestibular System.* 3rd ed. New York: Oxford University Press, 2001.

the debate was a better understanding of what was being tested with the different caloric methodologies. When the caloric test is performed with the patient fixating on a target, the observed nystagmus response is due to activation of the horizontal canal ocular reflex and the visual pursuit system. The latter generates a visual tracking movement in the opposite direction of the vestibular slow phase suppressing the nystagmus. Thus, the caloric test performed in the traditional method proposed by Hallpike is not a vestibular test but, rather, a test of the vestibular and visual pursuit systems combined. A more logical way to perform the test would be to measure the induced nystagmus with the eyes open in darkness (using the electronystagmographic system illustrated in Figure 15.3) to test the vestibulo-ocular reflex in isolation and then to turn on the lights and have the patient fixate to test the combined visual–vestibular response. Of course, electrical methods for recording eye movements were not available in 1942 when Fitzgerald and Hallpike originally reported their technique for performing the bithermal caloric test, but years later when such recording techniques were widely available, Hallpike stubbornly resisted any change in his caloric test methodology (Hallpike, 1975).

References

Bauer J, Leidler R. Über den Einfluß der Ausschaltung verschiedener Hirnabschnitte auf die vestibulären Augenreflexe. *Arb Neurol Inst Wien Univ* 1912;19:155–226.

Carmichael EA, Dix MR, Hallpike CS, et al. Some further observations upon the effect of unilateral cerebral lesions on caloric and rotational nystagmus. *Brain* 1961;84:571.

Cawthorne TE, Fitzgerald G, Hallpike CS. Observations on directional preponderance of caloric nystagmus resulting from unilateral labyrinthectomy. *Brain* 1942;56:138.

Dusser de Barenne JG, de Kleyn A. Ueber vestikulare augenreflexe v. vestibulartersuchungen nach ausschaltung einer grosshimhemisphare beim kaninchen. *Arch Ophthalmol Berlin* 1923;11:374–392.

Fitzgerald G, Hallpike CS. Studies in human vestibular function: 1. Observations on the directional preponderance ("Nystagmusbereitschaft") of caloric nystagmus resulting from cerebral lesions. *Brain* 1942;65:115–137.

Hakas P, Kornhuber H. Der vestibuläre Nystagmus bei Grosshirnläsionen des Menschen. *Arch Psychiatr Nervenkt* 1959;200:19.

Hallpike CS. Directional preponderance 1942–1974: A review. *Acta Otolaryngol* 1975;79:409–418.

Hoagland H. Quantitative analysis of responses from lateral line nerves of fishes: II. *J Gen Physiol* 1933;16:715–732.

Kobrak F. Berträge zum experimentellen Nystagmus. *Beitr Anat & c, Ohr* 1918;10:214.

Ledoux A. Les canaux semicirculaires. *Acta Otorinolaryngol Belg* 1958;12:109.

Löwenstein O, Sand A. The activity of the horizontal semicircular canal of the dogfish *Scyllium canicula. J Exp Biol* 1936;13:416.

Magnus R. *Körperstellung*. Berlin: Springer-Verlag, 1924.

Stahle J. Endolymphatic hydrops—Fiftieth anniversary. *Acta Otolaryngol (Stockh)* 1989;Suppl 468:11–16.

Hallpike Defines the Syndrome of Benign Paroxysmal Positional Vertigo

In 1952, Hallpike and his young assistant, Margaret Dix, published a landmark paper in neurotology titled "The Pathology, Symptomatology and Diagnosis of Certain Common Disorders of the Vestibular System." The paper was jointly published in the *Proceedings of the Royal Society of Medicine* and, in the United States, in the *Annals of Otology, Rhinology and Laryngology* (Dix and Hallpike, 1952a, 1952b). In the paper, they described the clinical profile of three of the most common causes of vertigo—Ménière's disease, vestibular neuronitis, and benign paroxysmal positional vertigo (BPPV). Their strategy was simple. First, identify the symptoms and natural history of the disease, then document the physical signs associated with the disease, and finally, whenever the opportunity presented itself, correlate the clinical features with histological studies of the temporal bones.

Dix was one of Hallpike's most faithful and devoted co-workers in the otologic unit at Queen Square. During World War II, Dix suffered severe facial cuts and lost vision in one eye when she was hit by flying glass from a bomb that struck the hospital where she was doing her surgical training. She went through a difficult period medically and emotionally, and it was doubtful if she would even be able to continue with a career in surgery, but she gained her surgical fellowship in 1943. Hallpike offered her a position along with J. D. Hood, a young physics graduate, in his newly formed Otological Research Unit in 1944. Their role at that time was to define the requirements for a mass-produced hearing aid that had become one of the priorities of the British Medical Research Council and an important consideration in the establishment of the new Otological Research Unit.

Dix and Hallpike developed a unique and productive working relationship. He went out of his way to protect her from any adverse clinical consequences due to her disability. She in turn acted as his legs, searching out the endless necessary books and journals from different libraries in that pre-copying era. Hallpike insisted on an alphabetical authorship that put Dix ahead of him in the published work of the Unit.

For her part, Dix idolized Hallpike. In her eyes, he could do no wrong. In a brief obituary published in *Nature* after Hallpike's death in 1979, Dix (1980) noted that

> Hallpike had the great merit of having inspired many collaborators to engage in scientific work and his wisdom and shrewd judgment will be remembered the world over. He was the acknowledged master of his subject, albeit a hard one, a perfectionist, utterly single-minded in all he undertook. He was quick to recognize and appreciate good work, intolerant of fools but unfailing in giving due credit to his co-workers. The fact that the majority of his unit staff remained with him over the years, a number from its inception until his retirement, is testimony in itself to his integrity. (p. 836)

Dix went on to have a productive career on her own after Hallpike retired from the Otologic Institute in 1965. She is probably best known for her work in developing vestibular exercises for rehabilitation of patients after acute vestibular injuries.

Clinical Features of BPPV

In their 1952 paper, Dix and Hallpike provided the first clinical description of the syndrome of BPPV. Since Bárány's description of the young woman with paroxysmal positional nystagmus in 1921 (see Chapter 11), numerous authors had attempted to classify positional nystagmus, but the subject had only become more confusing. As a starting point, Dix and Hallpike described the clinical features of a large number of cases they had seen in the Queen Square clinic. The characteristic history was that of a patient who developed brief episodes of vertigo when turning over in bed or getting in and out of bed or when changing position during the workday, such as "lying down beneath a car or in throwing the head backward to paint a ceiling." The patient usually recognized that the vertigo was associated with a critical position and would do his or her best to avoid that position. The vertigo could be accompanied by nausea and vomiting, but there were typically no other symptoms; specifically, hearing was usually normal.

They used a standard positioning technique to elicit the positional nystagmus (Figure 16.1) (Dix and Hallpike, 1952a):

> The patient is laid supine upon a couch with his head just over its end. The head is then lowered about 30° below the level of the couch and turned some 30 to 45° to one side. In taking up this position, the patient is first seated upon the couch with the head turned to one side and the gaze fixed upon the examiner's forehead. The examiner then grasps the patient's head firmly between his hands and briskly pushes the patient back into the critical position. (p. 349)

After a latent period of 5 or 6 seconds, the positional nystagmus begins:

> The onset of the nystagmus is nearly always preceded by an appearance of distress. The color may change; the patients may close their eyes, cry out in alarm and make active efforts to sit up again. At this point it is necessary to reassure the patient and maintain the position of the head. The nystagmus is chiefly rotatory (torsional), the direction of the rotation being toward the undermost ear. (p. 349)

Here, Dix and Hallpike had a note indicating that the direction of rotation is made in reference to the displacement of the 12 o'clock point of the corneal circumference. They went on to state,

> In addition to the rotatory element there is generally a horizantal component which is again directed toward the undermost ear. The

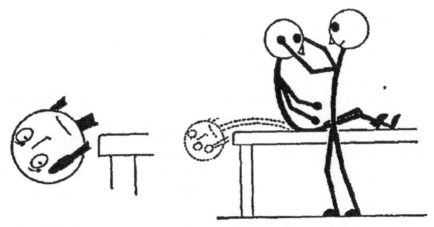

Figure 16.1 SCHEMATIC ILLUSTRATION OF THE DIX–HALLPIKE POSITIONAL TEST FOR BPPV. Source: From Dix MR, Hallpike CS. The pathology, symptomatology and diagnosis of certain common disorders of the vestibular system. *Proc R Soc Med* 1952;45:341–354.

nystagmus increases in a rapid crescendo in a period that may be as short as two-thirds of a second or as long as 10 seconds. Thereafter it rapidly declines and the patient's distress is relieved. If the patient is then allowed to sit up, a recurrence of the vertigo in a slighter form is generally noted, and if the eyes are examined at this point nystagmus can be seen, the direction of which is, on the whole, reversed. If this is allowed to disappear and the critical supine position is again assumed, the nystagmus again makes its appearance but generally in slighter form and disappears more rapidly than before. After two or three repetitions of this test it is generally found that the reaction has been eliminated altogether and cannot be elicited except, as Barany pointed out, after a period of rest. (p. 349)

Dix and Hallpike (1952a, 1952b) added important details to Bárány's earlier description. They emphasized the typical position changes that trigger the nystagmus and the benign course of the disorder. They induced the nystagmus on examination by briskly moving the patient from a sitting to head-hanging position, whereas Bárány simply turned the head to the side while the patient was lying supine. They identified a new feature not mentioned by Bárány—the latency period from the time of the position change to the onset of positional nystagmus. They also described a reversal in the positional nystagmus when the patient returned to the sitting position from the head-hanging position. Like Bárány, they noted that the nystagmus was chiefly rotatory (torsional), with the upper pole of the eye beating toward the ground. Also like Bárány, they noted that the nystagmus fatigued with repeated positioning only to recur after a period of rest.

Confusion Regarding the Direction of the Positional Nystagmus

There was one important inconsistency between the description of Dix and Hallpike and Bárány's original description. Dix and Hallpike (1952a, 1952b) noted that in addition to the rotatory (torsional) component, there was generally a horizontal component that was directed toward the undermost ear. Bárány, on the other hand, described the nystagmus as having a rotatory and vertical component, with the magnitude of the rotatory and vertical components changing with different positions of the eyes in the orbits (see Figure 11.3). Although Dix and Hallpike made no mention of this discrepancy in their paper, they had to be aware of it because they translated parts of Bárány's original paper, including the part that described the nystagmus direction. Their translation of the sentence from Bárány's paper describing the nystagmus direction read as follows: "When she did this, there appeared a strong rotatory nystagmus to the right." The actual sentence from Bárány's paper read, "When she did this, there appeared a strong rotatory nystagmus to the right with a vertical component upwards, which when looking to the right was purely rotatory, and when looking to the left was purely vertical" (Bárány, 1921; as translated by Lanska and Remler, 1997, p. 1168). Thus, in their translation, Dix and Hallpike left out the part of the sentence describing the vertical component of nystagmus. One can only assume that they did not agree with Bárány's observation and, therefore, decided to leave it out of their translation rather than indicating he was wrong. The irony of the situation is that Bárány was correct and they were wrong. In fact, Bárány's observation on the direction of the nystagmus and its changing rotatory and vertical components in different gaze directions was a key observation regarding the mechanism of the nystagmus. As discussed later, it indicated that the nystagmus originated from the posterior semicircular canal.

Strong Evidence for an Inner Ear Origin

Dix and Hallpike went on to describe the clinical details of 100 cases they evaluated who had typical benign paroxysmal positional nystagmus. They again emphasized the essentially benign course of the condition, noting that they had followed many of the cases for more than 5 years and in nearly all, the symptoms had spontaneously subsided. They noted, "all of our cases have been investigated by our neurological colleagues and, with one or two exceptions of doubtful significance, no evidence has been found of any neurological lesion. On the other hand evidence of associated ear disease was common" (Dix and Hallpike, 1952a, p. 351). Of the 100 cases, 55 were considered to have substantial evidence of ear disease, most commonly infections or trauma. Of the 55 cases with associated ear disease, the process was bilateral in 31 and unilateral in 24. In 21 of the 24 cases with unilateral ear disease, the positional nystagmus was induced when the abnormal ear was undermost—that is, facing toward the ground.

Many of their subjects complained of neck and occipital pain likely due to cervical arthritis, but they dismissed this as a possible etiologic factor because none of the patients had other neurological symptoms or signs. They also considered the possibility of a vascular disorder, possibly related to some underlying vascular abnormality. They noted that De Kleyn and Nieuwenhuyse (1927) had suggested the possibility that positional vertigo could result from occlusion of a vertebral artery within its bony canal in the neck because it could be shown that a vertebral artery may be occluded by certain head positions, particularly

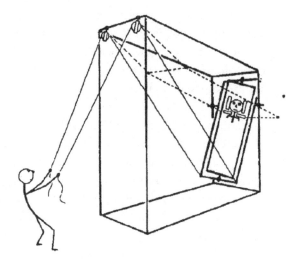

Figure 16.2 DEVICE DEVELOPED BY HALLPIKE AND COLLEAGUES TO POSITION
PATIENTS BACK INTO A HEAD-HANGING POSITION WITHOUT HAVING TO MOVE
THE NECK. Source: From Dix MR, Hallpike CS. The pathology, symptomatology and diagnosis of
certain common disorders of the vestibular system. *Proc R Soc Med* 1952;45:341–354.

the kind that commonly elicit benign paroxysmal positional nystagmus. To further assess this possibility, they designed an elaborate apparatus using ropes and
pulleys for positioning the patient into the critical head-back position without
bending the neck (Figure 16.2). With this apparatus, they were able to show
that the characteristic positional nystagmus occurred in the critical position
even though the neck position remained rigid throughout the entire positioning
process. Their final conclusion was that "the lesion is a peripheral one and in the
labyrinth towards which, when undermost, the nystagmus is directed" (Dix and
Hallpike, 1952a, p. 351). Regarding the nature of the lesion, they dismissed the
possibility of a tumor or hydrops considering the nature of the vertigo and the
benign course. Because the caloric responses were often normal, they concluded
that the process was likely irritative rather than destructive.

Pathology of BPPV

The coup de grace was a clinical–pathological correlation in a patient who developed BPPV prior to her death from a central nervous system glioma (tumor).
The patient had a 20-year history of right-sided deafness and recurrent vertigo,
and examination a few months before her death documented severe deafness
in the right ear, normal caloric responses on both sides, and benign paroxysmal positional nystagmus when the right ear was undermost. On histological

examination of the inner ears, the left inner ear was completely normal, but the right inner ear showed a severe degeneration of the spiral ganglion in the cochlea and degeneration of the otolith organs of the utricle and saccule. The ampullae of the semicircular canals were normal. The otolith organ of the utricle on the abnormal side showed an absence of the otolithic membrane, disorganization of the sensory cells, and considerable thickening of the subendothelial connective tissue with irregular cellular infiltrations. They concluded that these changes most likely were the result of either infection or trauma, consistent with their clinical impression that BPPV was commonly associated with infection or trauma of the inner ear. Their final conclusion was "that positional nystagmus of the benign paroxysmal type, first described by Barany in 1921, is due, as Barany believed, to otolith disease" (Dix and Hallpike, 1952a, p. 354).

In 1957, Hallpike and Terence Cawthorne, the senior ear, nose, and throat surgeon at Queen Square, reported a second clinical–pathological correlation of a case of BPPV. This patient had the typical clinical syndrome, but the interpretation was somewhat complicated because of metastatic carcinoma including multiple small metastases to the cerebellum. They effectively argued that the carcinoma was probably incidental, and the histological sections of the temporal bone again showed degeneration of the utricular otolith organ on the side that was undermost when the positional nystagmus was induced. In addition, this case showed degeneration of the crista of the horizontal semicircular canal on the same side, which they assumed was probably due to the same pathological mechanism that caused the utricular damage. Because there were atherosclerotic changes in the arteries of the brainstem and cerebellum, they speculated that these degenerative changes in the inner ear resulted from localized occlusion of the vascular supply to the inner ear. They argued that the paroxysmal positional nystagmus was triggered by the positional stimulus to a damaged but still functioning utricular otolith organ.

Final Years

Hallpike provided convincing evidence that BPPV originated from the inner ear when two patients with BPPV and a deaf ear were cured of the positional nystagmus after a chemical labyrinthectomy of the deaf ear. Along with his research-fellow Lewis Citron, Hallpike opened the horizontal semicircular canal, removed the membranous canal, and injected 95% alcohol into the inner ear (Citron and Hallpike, 1956). A third case of BPPV was cured after sectioning of the eighth cranial nerve (Citron and Hallpike, 1962). There were a few loose ends to the explanation that the paroxysmal positional nystagmus originated from a partially damaged utricular otolith organ, however. In the case reported in 1952, the utricular otolith organ was completely degenerated on the damaged side. Some utricular otolith function must remain in order to generate the abnormal positional response. More bothersome was the fact that no one had ever shown that a burst of nystagmus could be triggered from stimulation of an otolith organ. It had been a general dictum since the time of Lorente de Nó that nystagmus could only originate from the semicircular canal–ocular reflexes.

Hallpike refused to give up on his theory of an otolith origin for BPPV even though the evidence was heavily mounting against it. His final comments on positional nystagmus were presented at a meeting of the Barany Society in London in 1977 when he was 77 years old (Hallpike, 1978). By that time, Harold Schuknecht had proposed his cupulolithiasis mechanism for BPPV (see Chapter 17) and Richard Gacek had shown that selectively cutting the nerve from the posterior semicircular canal stopped the nystagmus. Hallpike acknowledged that these were weighty arguments for a posterior semicircular canal origin of the positional nystagmus, but he argued that the characteristics of the nystagmus indicated that it must arise from activation of several canals rather than a single canal. He believed that Schuknecht's explanation was less than complete, and he was unwilling to accept the fact that the nystagmus cannot be produced by the utricular otolith organ. He also believed that the condition might not be entirely dependent on peripheral mechanisms. Some features of the nystagmus he believed suggested a central mechanism. However, such remarks need to be interpreted in the context of his failing health by that time. His attendance at that meeting was in itself a formidable undertaking. He had suffered several transient ischemic attacks and had to give up driving in 1976 after having several minor accidents (as he stated, "when my thinking distance had reached half a mile") (Jeremy Hallpike, personal communication, 1998). Charles Hallpike died in Southampton on September 26, 1979, at the age of 79.

References

Bárány R. Diagnose von Krankheitserscheinungen im Bereiche des Otolithenapparates. *Acta Otolaryngol* 1921;2:434–437.

Cawthorne TE, Hallpike CS. A study of the clinical features and pathological changes within the temporal bones, brain stem and cerebellum of an early case of positional nystagmus of the so-called benign paroxysmal type. *Acta Otolaryngol* 1957;48:89–105.

Citron L, Hallpike CS. Observations upon the mechanism of positional nystagmus of the so-called "benign paroxysmal type." *J Laryngol Otol* 1956;70:253–259.

Citron L, Hallpike CS. A case of positional nystagmus of the so-called benign paroxysmal type and the effects of treatment by intracranial division of the VIIIth nerve. *J Laryngol Otol* 1962;76:28–33.

De Kleyn A, Nieuwenhuyse AC. Schwindelanflle und Nystagmus bei einer bestimmten Stellung des Kopfes. *Acta Otolaryngologica* 1927;11:155–157.

Dix MR. C. S. Hallpike. *Nature* 1980;284(5754):836.

Dix MR, Hallpike CS. The pathology, symptomatology and diagnosis of certain common disorders of the vestibular system. *Proc R Soc Med* 1952a;45:341–354.

Dix MR, Hallpike CS. The pathology, symptomatology and diagnosis of certain common disorders of the vestibular system. *Ann Otol Rhinol Layngol* 1952b;61:987.

Hallpike CS. Positional nystagmus. Some introductory remarks. In *Vestibular Mechanisms in Health and Disease: VI. Extraordinary meeting of the Barany Society.* Hood JD, ed. Academic Press: London, 1978, pp 167–177.

Lanska DJ, Remler B. Benign paroxysmal positional vertigo: Classic descriptions, origins of the provocative positioning technique, and conceptual developments. *Neurology* 1997;48:1167-1177.

SECTION 5

HAROLD SCHUKNECHT (1917–1996)

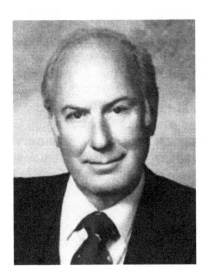

By the mid-20th century, the inner ear origin of benign paroxysmal positional vertigo (BPPV) was well established, but there was confusion regarding the appearance and origin of the characteristic nystagmus. Bárány and Hallpike both believed that the nystagmus originated from the gravity-sensing otolith organs, even though nystagmus was considered a semicircular canal–ocular reflex. Harold Schuknecht focused attention on the posterior semicircular canal after he observed that this was the only semicircular canal remaining in postmortem specimens from a few patients with BPPV. He speculated that otolithic debris, dislodged from the utricular otolith organ, became attached to the cupula of the posterior semicircular canal, making it sensitive to gravity—the cupulolithiasis model. Although Schuknecht's model did not account for all of the features of BPPV, it provided the framework for our current understanding of the disorder.

Schuknecht and His Breakthrough on Benign Paroxysmal Positional Vertigo

John Lindsay and the University of Chicago Otology Clinic

In 1928, John Lindsay arrived at the newly established Medical Center at the University of Chicago as an assistant professor in the Division of Otolaryngology (Marion, 1983; Schuknecht, 1983). Lindsay grew up on a farm in Ontario, Canada, attended a 6-year medical program at McGill University, and then entered private practice in the office of a country doctor. He quickly realized that he did not know enough about medicine to be effective with most of his patients, so he decided to focus to one specialty, entering a residency in otolaryngology first at the University of Toronto and then at McGill University. With the support of Dallas Phemister, Chief of Surgery, a year of sabbatical leave was arranged so that Lindsay could visit Europe to learn the latest developments in otological surgery. He spent most of the time in Zurich, Switzerland, working with F. R. Nager, Chief of Otolaryngology at the University of Zurich.

In the tradition of Wittmaack, Nager had his practice in a small house just down the hill from the university buildings. His patient examination rooms were next door to his research laboratory. Nager had learned the art of processing temporal bones and began to develop his own temporal bone library. Lindsay was given a desk in the laboratory and was called next door to the examination rooms whenever Nager had a patient he believed Lindsay should see. In this setting, Lindsay became fascinated with the study of temporal bone pathology. He watched the technician process and cut the bones, and he routinely reviewed the histological sections with Nager. When Lindsay returned from Europe, he was offered a position at the University of Chicago, where he established a temporal bone research program of his own. Lindsay stated (as quoted in Marion, 1983),

When I got back from Europe, I started to save, from the morgue, every ear I could get my hands on—or anybody else could get their hands on. The processing took about a year after you got the ears; then you could study what was going on. (p. 10)

At that time, a debate was beginning regarding whether biomedical research should be relegated to full-time basic researchers or whether physicians in clinical practice had a role to play. Lindsay believed that physicians knew the clinical expressions of disease and therefore were best able to establish and maintain a relationship between clinical medicine and research. He recruited several like-minded physicians on the Otolaryngology faculty, and he insisted that his resident physicians were exposed to research during their training (Schuknecht, 1983). On the other hand, he was well aware of the competing forces of the need to make a living (as quoted in Marion, 1983):

Some people are naturally interested in doing high quality research, making a reputation through what they do, what they produce, then there are others who get their satisfaction out of making money. There seem to be two sets of ideals, one set being for those who make the big money and just can't resist it. Money is useful, of course, but it is much more satisfying to go after knowledge. (p. 11)

Schuknecht Begins His Residency at the University of Chicago

In this fertile environment, Harold Schuknecht, who had recently returned from the war in Europe, began his residency training in January 1946. While stationed in Italy, Schuknecht had enjoyed his work in an eye clinic and decided to apply for an eye residency after he returned to the United States. When he attempted to apply to the eye, ear, nose, and throat residency at the University of Chicago, he was told that during the war, the eye residency program had separated from the ear, nose, and throat (ENT) program. All of the eye residency positions were full, but there was still a position in ENT. He decided to take the position because he did not want to delay his residency training. Prior to coming to the University of Chicago, Schuknecht had no formal exposure to research and planned on a career in the private practice of surgery. He soon came under the influence of John Lindsay and also Henry Perlman and Heinrich Kohr, who were young academic-oriented otolaryngologists recruited by Lindsay in the early 1930s and who, along with Lindsay, formed the backbone of the Otolaryngology Division (Fernandez, 1983).

During his residency, Schuknecht examined the temporal bone specimens from several patients who had suffered severe head injuries and noted a characteristic pattern of cochlear damage primarily involving the basilar turn of the cochlea (Schuknecht, 1950). This led to his first series of scientific experiments in which he tested hearing and examined the cochlea for damage after delivering blows to the exposed skull of anesthetized cats (Schuknecht et al., 1951). In collaboration with William Neff, an experimental psychologist, Schuknecht developed a method to obtain pure tone hearing thresholds in the animals using behavioral methods (Neff, 1984). After the blows to the head, he found that the cochlear damage was greatest in the upper basal turn and that the hearing loss affected a greater range of frequencies as the cochlear damage became more widespread. This first experimental study, which was published in *The Annals of Otology, Rhinology, and Laryngology* in 1950, stimulated Schuknecht's interest in the relationship between the locus of cochlear damage and the frequencies for which hearing loss occurred. In order to conduct his research during his busy surgical residency, Schuknecht did most of his experiments in the evening and on weekends. Basic researchers were amazed to see this young surgeon testing hearing in cats late into the evenings (Kiang, 1984).

Schuknecht's Formative Years

In many ways, Harold Schuknecht is the prototypical American success story. He was born in a small farming community in Chancellor, South Dakota, in 1917 (Nadol, 1997). His father, also born in South Dakota, quit school after the sixth grade to work on the family farm. Despite his lack of education, his father was known for his knack with numbers, being able to add long columns in his head. His paternal grandfather was also a farmer who migrated to South Dakota from a German community in Wisconsin. He had no formal education and had never learned to read. Schuknecht's mother's family came to South Dakota from Germany when she was 4 years old. They were Baptist fundamentalists who left Germany in part because of religious persecution. Schuknecht's early family life was dominated by his mother's strong fundamentalist beliefs. She regularly attended prayer meetings, and the entire family was expected to attend Sunday services and Sunday school. Harold's father had to stop playing baseball in a semi-pro league because she did not allow him to play on Sundays. Every morning, the family gathered together and Harold's father read a section from the Bible, the only book in the house (Anne Schuknecht, Harold Schuknecht's wife, personal communication, 1998).

Harold worked on the farm from morning to night, 6 days a week, except for the time that he was at school. He developed a work ethic that would stay with him throughout his life. The family was extremely poor, and it was in constant danger of losing the farm during the Depression years. His father took on an additional job operating a grain elevator in town to earn enough money to make the mortgage payments on the farm. He expected Harold to stay and take over the farm as he had done with his father's farm, but Harold's mother encouraged him to go to college so that he could become a teacher. Harold made his choice on a hot dusty summer day in the middle of a prolonged drought period. He was following behind five horses dragging a field that had just been plowed when he decided that this was not what he wanted to do for the rest of his life (Anne Schuknecht, personal communication, 1998).

Schuknecht enrolled at the University of South Dakota in 1934. At that time, the tuition was $35 a semester, a major factor in his choice of schools. He chose pre-med as a major because a friend of his from high school, and his roommate at the university, had chosen pre-med as a major. The two young doctors-to-be were able to obtain a room rent-free from a retired doctor in return for helping him around the house (boyhood friend Dave Dahlin, personal communication, 1998). Their only expense was an average of $2 a week for food for the two of them. For entertainment, they played handball and swam in the school pool, and occasionally on weekends they would sneak into the local movie theater.

Schuknecht began medical school in 1936 after cramming 3 years of premedical training into 2 years by attending summer classes. The tuition in medical school increased to $50 a semester, so Schuknecht had to work several part-time jobs to meet his increased payments. Only the first 2 years of medical school were offered at the University of South Dakota, so he had to apply to another medical school for the final 2 years. He was accepted at Rush Medical College at the University of Chicago, but this meant a dramatic jump in tuition to $450 a year. With his father's help, he was able to arrange a loan through a cousin that he paid back with interest over several years after he finished his medical training (Anne Schuknecht, personal communication, 1998). He graduated from Rush Medical College in 1940 and then spent a year doing a rotating internship at Mercy Hospital in Des Moines, Iowa. On his first day of work, he met his wife-to-be, Anne Bodle, who had just come to work at the hospital as a laboratory technician. They were married exactly 1 year later and had their first child, a daughter, 1 year after that.

With World War II intensifying, Schuknecht joined the reserves and he was soon called to active duty. After spending 2 years in the States, he spent 2 years as a flight surgeon with the 15th Air Force Division in the Mediterranean Theater. While stationed in Italy, he was in the first ambulance to arrive as a B-24 crashed during landing, setting off a fire and several explosions. All of the crew members were able to get out except for the pilot, who was trapped in the burning cockpit. Schuknecht climbed onto the plane, pulled him out, and rolled him on the ground to put out the fire. Soon after rescuing the pilot, the plane exploded.

For his heroics rescuing the pilot, Schuknecht received the Soldier's Medal. Schuknecht loved to fly, having obtained his pilot's license while stationed in the States. While in Europe, he frequently went on "milk runs" just for the fun of flying. The practice came to an abrupt end, however, when a routine "milk run" turned into a major battle with the Luftwaffe. The bomber next to his was shot down, and his plane barely made it back to the airfield (Dave Dahlin, personal communication, 1998).

After completing his residency in 1949, Schuknecht stayed on at the University of Chicago first as a clinical instructor and then as an assistant professor. His clinical activities were largely directed at general head and neck surgery and endoscopy, and he continued his experimental work on the relationship between the locus of cochlear damage and the frequencies of associated hearing loss. He made precise surgical lesions in different parts of the cochlea and carefully measured the effect on hearing after the animals had recovered (Schuknecht, 1953). Animals with lesions at the base of the cochlea showed a characteristic high-frequency hearing loss, whereas those with lesions at the apex developed a low-frequency hearing loss. He then conducted a series of experiments testing hearing in animals after lesions of the auditory nerve. He eventually developed a complete map of the cat's cochlea showing the relationship between hearing loss and locus of cochlear damage (Nadol, 1997).

Throughout his academic career, Schuknecht continued the rigorous work pattern established during his residency. His wife Anne learned to adjust. After their first child was born in 1942, Anne developed a severe case of rheumatoid arthritis and she was told that she would probably never be able to have more children. Remarkably, Anne had a spontaneous remission from her rheumatoid arthritis, and they had their second child, a son, in 1951. Anne spent her time caring for the children, and Harold spent his time developing his career (Anne Schuknecht, personal communication, 1998).

Despite the heavy surgical workload, Schuknecht was making less than $15,000 a year as a young assistant professor at the University of Chicago. Money began to be an issue because he was still repaying his medical school debts and he had a wife and two young children to provide for. Furthermore, he was concerned about raising young children, particularly a young daughter, in the rough neighborhood around the University of Chicago. When the opportunity of a higher paying position as Chief of Otolaryngology at Henry Ford Hospital in Detroit arose in 1953, he decided to take it even though he was unsure about what effect this might have on his promising academic career and the experimental research he was conducting at the University of Chicago. An unexpected benefit of the move to Henry Ford Hospital was that Schuknecht was able to focus his clinical activity on otological surgery and establish an experimental research laboratory on his own. At Henry Ford Hospital, he was in the forefront in developing new otological surgical techniques, including the development of stapedectomy surgery that revolutionized the management of otosclerosis. Throughout his career, he performed more than 1000 stapedectomy surgeries, gradually refining the technique (Anne Schuknecht, personal communication, 1998).

Schuknecht Becomes Interested in BPPV

On December 22, 1956, a 77-year-old woman was hospitalized at the Henry Ford Hospital because of severe recurrent attacks of vertigo (Schuknecht, 1962). These episodes typically occurred after turning over in bed, particularly when she turned onto her right side. After getting up, she had a sudden sensation of falling backward, which on one occasion caused her to fall and hit the back of her head. Her only other symptom was a progressive hearing loss in the right ear dating back many years. When Schuknecht examined the woman, he noted positional nystagmus when she was positioned with the right ear down, typical of the type seen with BPPV. After a brief latency, there was a burst of counterclockwise torsional nystagmus lasting 5 or 6 seconds. The nystagmus fatigued with repeated testing. She had a profound hearing loss in the right ear and a moderate hearing loss in the left ear. Schuknecht read Hallpike's report earlier that year of two cases of BPPV cured after a labyrinthectomy, so he performed a right labyrinthectomy on the woman, removing the inner ear through the oval window on December 19, 1956. After the operation, the vertigo and nystagmus were gone. This case convinced Schuknecht that BPPV originated from the inner ear and stimulated him to review the pathology of patients reported with BPPV, ultimately leading to his development of the cupulolithiasis theory for BPPV.

Search for the Cause of BPPV

In 1956, John Lindsay, along with one of his residents, Garth Hemenway, reported a 65-year-old woman who without any prior illnesses suddenly developed severe vertigo, nausea, and vomiting that gradually resolved over several weeks. Approximately 1 month after the onset of this acute prolonged episode of vertigo, she experienced brief recurrent attacks of positional vertigo, triggered by turning onto her right side while in bed or when getting in and out of bed. When examined, she had a bilateral sloping sensorineural hearing loss, slightly greater in the right ear, but she had not noticed any change in hearing with her vertigo symptoms. Positional testing triggered positional vertigo and nystagmus when she was turned onto her right side and when sitting up from the recumbent position (no description of the nystagmus was given). There was no response to caloric stimulation of the right ear, even with ice water. The patient died of a coronary thrombosis approximately 13 years after the acute prolonged vertigo episode, and on postmortem examination of the temporal bones, there was a remarkably selective degeneration of the superior division of the vestibular nerve and the sense organs supplied by it—the otolith organ (macule) of the utricle and cristae of the horizontal and anterior semicircular canals (see Figure 1.1).

In the same paper, Lindsay and Hemenway described an additional six cases with a similar clinical picture of acute vertigo followed by positional vertigo. They concluded that the cause of the acute prolonged vertigo in all of their cases was a vascular accident affecting the vestibular mechanism on one side. Regarding the delayed onset positional vertigo, they believed that it was unlikely to originate from the macule of the utricle (as proposed by Bárány and Hallpike) because the macule of the utricle was degenerated in the case they had studied postmortem. They concluded that the positional vertigo likely originated from the saccule or posterior canal because these were the only organs remaining intact (Lindsay and Hemenway, 1956).

Schuknecht reviewed the temporal bone specimens from the patient reported by his former mentor, John Lindsay, and from the patients reported by Hallpike and colleagues, and he was struck by the remarkable similarity in the pathologic changes (Schuknecht, 1962). Each had a selective degeneration of the superior part of the labyrinth, including the superior branch of the vestibular nerve, the utricle, and the cristae of the horizontal and superior semicircular canals. He concluded that in each case, the damage to the labyrinth resulted from occlusion of the anterior vestibular artery, the branch of the internal auditory artery that supplies the superior division of the vestibular nerve, the utricular macule, and the cristae of the posterior and anterior semicircular canals (Figure 17.1). Schuknecht believed that the delayed positional vertigo that occurred in these cases must have originated from the posterior semicircular canal because it was the only peripheral sensory organ capable of generating nystagmus that was still functioning. He dismissed the saccule as a possibility because it had never been shown to generate nystagmus.

With this hypothesis in mind, Schuknecht attempted to produce paroxysmal positional nystagmus in cats by cutting off the blood supply in the left anterior vestibular artery (Schuknecht, 1962). The superior division of the left vestibular nerve was cut along with the artery because it was not technically possible to block the artery alone. He studied four cats, and each developed the expected acute vestibular syndrome with horizontal nystagmus and imbalance in the immediate postoperative period. After these acute vestibular symptoms gradually subsided over several days, one of the animals developed typical benign paroxysmal positional nystagmus 3 months after the operation that persisted until

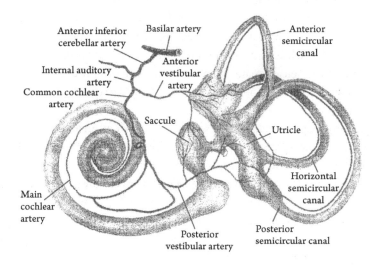

Figure 17.1 ARTERIAL BLOOD SUPPLY TO THE INNER EAR. Source: Courtesy Harold Schuknecht (1973).

termination of the experiment at 7 months. The animal exhibited a rotatory (torsional) clockwise nystagmus when placed in the supine position with the left ear undermost.

There was a latency and fatigability with repeated positioning. When the animal's temporal bones were examined 7 months after the operation, all showed severe atrophy of the superior division of the vestibular nerve and the sense organs supplied by that nerve. The posterior semicircular canal cristae and the inferior division of the vestibular nerve were intact. Thus, he was able to reproduce the clinical picture of an acute vertiginous syndrome followed by the delayed onset of positional nystagmus in one of four cats that underwent sectioning of the anterior vestibular artery. He speculated that collapse of the superior part of the inner ear might have interfered with the function of the posterior semicircular canal in the animals that did not develop positional nystagmus.

Schuknecht Suggests a New Mechanism for BPPV

Schuknecht presented the results of his studies on BPPV at the 66th annual session of the American Academy of Ophthalmology and Otolaryngology in October 1961 in Chicago. The paper was published in the *Transactions of the American Academy of Ophthalmology and Otolaryngology* the following year

(Schuknecht, 1962). Schuknecht effectively argued that based on his review of the human temporal bone specimens and his animal experiments, the only logical source for the paroxysmal positional nystagmus was the posterior semicircular canal. He reasoned that with degeneration of the superior vestibular labyrinth, otoconia would be released from the otolithic membrane of the utricular macule and that, in certain positions of the head, the otoconia would respond to gravity and thereby activate the cupula of the posterior semicircular canal (which sits directly below the utricular macule). The otoconia of the otolithic membrane are made of calcium carbonate that has a specific gravity of approximately 3. Its normal function is to render the macule gravity sensitive, thus providing the brain with information about the position of the head in space (see Figure 6.3). Schuknecht argued,

> It seems reasonable to assume that if released from the otolithic membrane, they might well persist for some time in the endolymph of the pars superior [utricle]. With the head in the erect position, the ampulla of the posterior canal lies in the most dependent portion of the pars superior, so it is in this region that any free particles of greater density than the endolymph would accumulate [Figure 17.2]. When the head is positioned for testing positional vertigo, that is, lowered 30 degrees below the level of the couch and turned some 30 to 45 degrees to one side, the posterior canal ampulla of the undermost ear is brought into a position superior to the utricle. From this position, the otoconia would be free to move downward into the utricle. The hypothesis assumes that the otoconia come to have a close relationship to the cupula of the posterior canal when the head is in the erect position, and when the ear is turned over, the downward movement of the otoconia creates a sharp ampullopetal (toward the utricle) deflection of the cupula. (pp. 328–329)

Schuknecht (1962) went on to explain how the otoconia hypothesis could account for the common clinical features of BPPV:

> The latent period, which usually is several seconds, may be due to the period of time required to get the otoconia into motion; the severity of the nystagmus may be due to the magnitude of the displacement of the cupula; the fatigability may be due to dispersing the crystals in the endolymph of the par superior during repeated head position changes; the short duration of the vertiginous attack may be due to the return of the cupula to its normal position after the otoconia have left it; the repeatability after rest may be due to the period of time needed for the

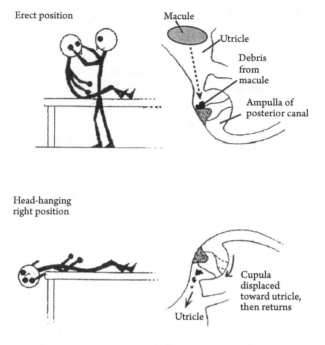

Figure 17.2 Schematic illustration of Schuknecht's original
theory for the production of benign paroxysmal positional
nystagmus. Source: From Schuknecht HF. *Pathology of the Ear.* Cambridge, Harvard
University Press, 1974.

otoconia to settle again into the posterior canal ampulla so that they
can again act en masse when the pars superior is turned over. (p. 329)

Schuknecht's key observation after reviewing the temporal bone specimens
from the three patients with BPPV was that the positional vertigo and nystagmus must originate from the posterior semicircular canal because it was the only
sense organ capable of generating nystagmus that remained. An important question that Schuknecht did not address in the 1962 paper was whether the appearance of the paroxysmal positional nystagmus was consistent with activation of
the posterior semicircular canal. If his hypothesis was correct, then the observed
positional nystagmus must be consistent with an ampullopetal deflection of the
cupula of the posterior semicircular canal that would result in an inhibition of
the spontaneous firing rate in the ampullary nerve from that canal.

Interestingly, in the introduction to his 1962 paper, Schuknecht provided a
translation of Bárány's original description of benign paroxysmal positional nystagmus from his 1921 paper. Like Dix and Hallpike, Schuknecht mentioned only
the rotatory component, leaving out the part of the sentence that described the
vertical component and the effect of gaze on the rotatory (torsional) and vertical

components. He presumably used the translation from the 1952 paper of Dix and Hallpike without checking the original reference. John Lindsay was asked to discuss Schuknecht's paper at the Academy meeting in 1961 (Lindsay, 1962). Lindsay acknowledged that Schuknecht's theory could simplify a complicated problem, but he rejected the theory because he thought it was too simple. He argued that there are many different types of positional nystagmus associated with many different ear diseases:

> It is a well established law that stimulation of any semicircular canal causes eye movements in the plane of that canal. Therefore, the variation in the plane and direction of the positional nystagmus which has been observed in many peripheral lesions seems to refute the theory of origin from the posterior canal. (p. 332)

Lindsay noted that a colleague at the University of Chicago, Cesar Fernandez, produced positional nystagmus of the paroxysmal type in cats when he ablated the nodular lobe of the cerebellum. Furthermore, this clear central type of positional nystagmus was abolished if the peripheral vestibular apparatus was destroyed. Therefore, the observation that benign paroxysmal positional nystagmus disappears after destruction of the peripheral labyrinth is not proof of a peripheral origin of the positional nystagmus. It could be a central type of positional nystagmus that requires peripheral input. Lindsay objected to the use of "benign" in describing the paroxysmal nystagmus because he argued that many central lesions that caused paroxysmal positional nystagmus were not benign. In support of his argument, he mentioned three cases of so-called benign paroxysmal positional nystagmus that turned out to be due to tumors of the cerebellar vermis. Lindsay had a way of presenting his comments in a constructive rather than a critical tone, always careful not to challenge or offend a colleague. Lindsay's criticisms reflected the general chaos in thinking about positional nystagmus at the time and were mostly wrong, but the fact that they were made by his former mentor strongly motivated Schuknecht to search for more compelling evidence for his new theory on BPPV.

References

Bárány R. Diagnose von Krankheitserscheinungen im Bereiche des Otolithenapparates. *Acta Otolaryngol* 1921;2:434–437.

Dix MR, Hallpike CS. The pathology, symptomatology and diagnosis of certain common disorders of the vestibular system. *Proc R Soc Med* 1952;45:341–354.

Fernandez C. Pioneers in research in otolaryngology at the University of Chicago. *Ann Otol Rhinol Laryngol* 1983;92(Suppl 102):23–26.

Kiang NYS. HFS: A personal perspective. *Ann Otol Rhinol Laryngol (Suppl)* 1984;112:142–144.

Lindsay JR. Discussion. *Trans Am Acad Ophthalmol Otol* 1962:331–332.

Lindsay JR, Hemenway WG. Postural vertigo due to unilateral sudden partial loss of vestibular function. *Ann Otol Rhinol Laryngol* 1956;65:692–706.

Marion M. Interviews with John Lindsay. *Ann Otol Rhinol Laryngol* 1983;92(Suppl 102):8–11.

Nadol JB. In memoriam: Harold F. Schuknecht, MD. *Am J Otol* 1997;18:133–135.

Neff WD. Harold Schuknecht: Beginnings of experimental research. *Ann Otol Rhinol Laryngol (Suppl)* 1984;112:9–11.

Schuknecht H. A clinical study of auditory damage following blows to the head. *Ann Otol Rhinol Laryngol* 1950;59:331–357.

Schuknecht HF. Techniques for study of cochlear function and pathology in experimental animals: Development of the anatomical frequency scale for the cat. *Arch Otolaryngol* 1953;58:177–397.

Schuknecht HF. Positional vertigo: Clinical and experimental observations. *Trans Am Acad Ophthalmol Otol* 1962:319–331.

Schuknecht HF. John Lindsay: Clinician, teacher, otopathologist. *Ann Otol Rhinol Laryngol* 1983;92(Suppl 102):12–16.

Schuknecht HF, Neff WD, Perlman HB. An experimental study of auditory damage following blows to the head. *Ann Otol Rhinol Laryngol* 1951;60:273–289.

Schuknecht's Temporal Bone
Bank in Boston

Harold Schuknecht was initially approached regarding the position of Chief of Otolaryngology at the Massachusetts Eye and Ear Infirmary at Harvard University in 1959, but he had just completed his new research laboratory at Henry Ford Hospital and he was uneasy about leaving even though the Harvard position was the opportunity of a lifetime (Anne Schuknecht, personal communication, 1998). Fortunately, Harvard was not able to decide on a new chief in 1959 and appointed an interim chief (Kiang, 1984). Two years later, Schuknecht reconsidered and took the position at Harvard.

When Schuknecht arrived at Harvard to chair the Department of Otolaryngology in 1961, he immediately set up a temporal bone laboratory and began collecting temporal bone specimens. His friend, Joseph Nadol (1997), later stated that

> it is safe to say that Schuknecht's main hobby was the temporal bone, and he took great joy and satisfaction in not only deriving knowledge of human otologic disease from the temporal bone, but in sharing it with his staff and trainees. He was known to have said that studying the temporal bone on Sunday morning was closer to religion than attending church services. (p. 135)

His "Sunday school" temporal bone sessions with the resident physicians were a regular feature of his early years as Chief of Otolaryngology at Harvard.

Without a doubt, Schuknecht was a workaholic. He typically left for work between 6:00 and 6:30 a.m. and did not return until after 7:30 p.m. Saturday was also a working day, although he usually left for work slightly later in the morning. Sunday was his leisure day; he usually spent only 4 hours in the hospital on Sunday. He worked on reading manuscripts and writing research papers when he was at home. He slept 5 or 6 hours a night at most but not infrequently would awaken early, as early as 2:00 a.m., particularly when he was working on his textbook, *Pathology of the Ear*. Schuknecht did not consider himself intellectually gifted, but he was proud of what he called his "intellectual stamina" (Anne Schuknecht, personal communication, 1998). He just worked harder and stuck with things longer than others.

Despite his heavy workload, Schuknecht maintained a fascination with sports. He had a lifelong interest in fishing and hiking that was spawned by his childhood in rural South Dakota. He took great pride in the Boston Marathon, regularly filming the runners and keeping detailed records on all of the marathons that he had seen. He liked to wait at the halfway point and encourage the runners who he knew. Every year, he held a party at his home for friends who participated in the marathon. Like most Americans, he had a fascination with the professional sports teams in his home city. He had season tickets to the Boston Celtics basketball games during the 1960s and 1970s when the Celtics dominated professional basketball. Joseph Nadol (1997) noted that

> one of his fondest memories and most prized trophies was catching the game ball after the final seventh game of the 1965 championship series with the Los Angeles Lakers when the ball was thrown into the stands by Sam Jones. The ball was subsequently autographed by all of the Celtics players and occupied a favorite spot in his den. (p. 135)

More Temporal Bone Specimens from Patients with Benign Paroxysmal Positional Vertigo

All three temporal bone specimens from patients with benign paroxysmal positional vertigo (BPPV) that Schuknecht reviewed in his 1962 paper showed degeneration of the superior part of the labyrinth (the anterior and horizon canals and the utricle) with sparing of the inferior part (the posterior canal and the saccule). However, as Dix and Hallpike (1952) noted, benign paroxysmal positional nystagmus usually occurs as an isolated finding without other damage to the inner ear. These cases, therefore, were not representative of the usual case of BPPV. In his Boston temporal bone laboratory, Schuknecht obtained two temporal bone specimens from patients with a more typical clinical picture of BPPV (Schuknecht, 1969). The first was a 69-year-old woman who experienced episodes of vertigo precipitated by stooping over, lying down, and most often when rolling onto the left side in bed. The episodes were of short duration, could be precipitated at will, and were not associated with auditory symptoms. Positional testing provoked a severe vertiginous episode of short duration associated with clockwise torsional nystagmus when she was placed in the supine left ear down position. Although details regarding latency, duration, and fatigability were not documented in the record, this appeared to be a case of typical BPPV. Hearing was normal for her age, and caloric responses were normal bilaterally. These symptoms persisted and were last documented at age 74, 3 years prior to her death of a massive cerebral hemorrhage at age 77.

The second patient was a 64-year-old woman who experienced brief episodes of positional vertigo typically triggered by turning over onto her left side or when getting out of bed. On positional testing, she exhibited a clockwise torsional nystagmus with the head in the left ear down position. In this case it was documented that there was a 6-second latency, a duration of 7 seconds, and there a reversal of the torsional nystagmus with return to the upright position. Again, auditory testing and caloric responses were normal. The episodes of positional vertigo continued unchanged for 4 years when, at age 68, the patient suddenly died of a pulmonary embolus.

In the temporal bone specimens from these two patients, Schuknecht identified a prominent granular basophilic staining mass attached to the cupula of the left posterior semicircular canal (Figure 18.1). There was also a thin layer of similar material located on the membranous wall of the posterior semicircular canal in its most inferior location in the second case only. Schuknecht did not find similar material, either attached to the cupula or on the membranous wall of

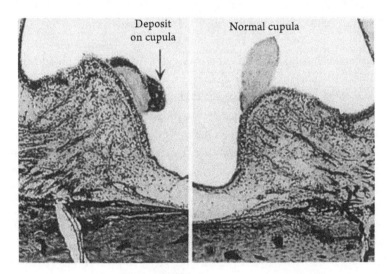

Figure 18.1 HISTOLOGICAL SECTIONS SHOWING BASOPHILIC DEPOSIT ON THE CUPULA OF THE LEFT POSTERIOR SEMICIRCULAR CANAL AND NORMAL CUPULA ON THE RIGHT OF A PATIENT WHO EXHIBITED TYPICAL BENIGN PAROXYSMAL POSITIONAL NYSTAGMUS IN THE HEAD-HANGING LEFT POSITION PRIOR TO DEATH FROM UNRELATED CAUSES. The cupula has shrunk due to postmortem artifact. Source: From Schuknecht HF. *Pathology of the Ear.* Cambridge, Harvard University Press, 1974.

the posterior semicircular canal, on the right side (the normal side). The macule of the utricle and saccule and also the three cristae of the semicircular canals were completely normal in both ears from both specimens.

The nature of this basophilic deposit that was located on the cupula of the posterior canal was not clear, but Schuknecht believed that it was probably derived from otoconia that had been detached from the otolithic membrane of the macule. Calcium would have been resorbed during the decalcification process, so he assumed that it was the matrix in which the calcium carbonate was embedded that stained with hematoxylin (a commonly used dye for staining postmortem tissue). It was also possible that the deposits represented products of degeneration from other sources. He mentioned that in a study of 550 specimens at the Massachusetts Eye and Ear Infirmary examined by his associate, Ralph Ruby, similar deposits on the cupulae of the posterior canals were found in only 15, and he suggested that some of these deposits might have resulted from postmortem degeneration of the utricular macule.

The Cupulolithiasis Theory

Based on the findings in the two previously mentioned postmortem specimens, Schuknecht (1969) coined the term "cupulolithiasis" ("stones on the cupula") to explain the clinical syndrome of BPPV. He assumed that

> substances having a specific gravity greater than endolymph and thus subject to movement with changes in the direction of gravitational force come into contact with the cupula of the posterior semicircular canal. Presumably, these particles may exist free in the endolymph or may become attached to the cupula. With the head in the erect position, the posterior canal ampulla is located inferiorly, whereas in the provocative test position (supine, head hanging, ear down), the posterior canal assumes a superior position. (p. 123)

As in his 1962 paper, Schuknecht (1969) believed that the limited duration of the vertiginous attacks resulted from "the return of the cupula to a normal position after the particles have left it" (p. 123), so even though he used the term cupulolithiasis, he was aware that the mass must float away from the cupula when the critical position was reached or otherwise the cupula would stay deviated and the positional nystagmus would not be of a short duration. Fatigability could be explained on the basis of dispersion of the particles in the endolymph, and repeatability after rest could be explained by the particles again settling into the posterior canal ampulla so that they could again act en masse when the critical position was achieved.

Schuknecht emphasized the benign nature of the disorder that he called cupulolithiasis and that the diagnosis could be readily made at the bedside with the provocative positioning test described by Dix and Hallpike (1952). He concluded that "the most rational and most simple management of the disorder is avoidance of the provocative position, and most patients accomplish this with little restriction of normal every day activities" (Schuknecht, 1969, p. 124). He suggested that the amount of restrictions depended on the characteristics of the attacks, such as suddenness of onset, severity of disequilibrium, associated nausea and vomiting, and frequency of occurrence. He suggested that climbing, swimming, and athletic activities such as skiing might be contraindicated and that operation of mechanical equipment such as driving an automobile or tending industrial machinery might have to be curtailed. His experience had shown that when BPPV followed head injury or ear surgery, it tended to remit within a few weeks or months, but when it was secondary to ear infection, aging, or vascular occlusion, it could be more persistent: "The precise symptoms and course probably are determined in a large degree by the physical characteristics of the cupular deposit—for example, the mass, specific gravity, solubility, and whether it is free or fixed to the cupula" (p. 124). He believed that it was a rare case in which the disability was so severe that a surgical procedure to ablate the vestibular labyrinth was justified.

Schuknecht Was Not the First to Propose the Cupulolithiasis Theory

Although the cupulolithiasis theory for the generation of BPPV is generally attributed to Schuknecht, he was not the first to consider this mechanism. As noted previously, Karl Wittmaack performed a series of experiments on guinea pigs in 1909 during which he rotated them at a very high speed, dislodging the heavy otolithic membrane from the macules of the utricle and saccule. On histological examination, Wittmaack noted pieces of the otolithic membrane scattered throughout the inner ear. In a comment on a paper published by Nylen on positional nystagmus in *Acta Otolaryngologica* in 1927, Wittmaack noted,

> In guinea pigs whose otolithic membrane has been rotated off you can sometimes observe a sudden nystagmus with changes of head position. This phenomenon occurred only when the otolith membrane was lying on or adjacent to the cupula, so that the phenomenon was undoubtedly explained by a pathological loading of the cupula with the otolithic membrane. Therefore, the possibility of a such a loading with concretions or something similar has to be considered as an explanation for

this phenomenon in certain cases [particularly when the origin is post-traumatic]. (p. 156)

These experiments were never published because they were never completed due to World War I. Harold Schuknecht apparently was unaware of Wittmaack's brief comment that was published in German.

A Key Question: Which Way Does the Cupula Deviate?

In his 1969 paper, Schuknecht concluded that movement of the head from the erect position to the provocative head-hanging position (with the standard Dix–Hallpike positional test) would result in an ampullofugal (away from the utricle) displacement of the cupula of the posterior semicircular canal due to the cupulolithiasis, whereas in his 1962 paper, he had concluded that the critical position change would result in an ampullopetal (toward the utricle) displacement of the cupula of the posterior semicircular canal (see Figure 17.2). This confusion regarding the expected direction of the cupular deviation with his cupulolithiasis theory would continue to haunt Schuknecht. Solving this puzzle (by others) ultimately led to an understanding of the mechanism of BPPV and a simple cure.

How to Explain the Stereotypical Nystagmus

While Schuknecht was preparing his 1969 paper on cupulolithiasis, he received a prepublication draft of a paper describing the stereotyped appearance of benign paroxysmal positional nystagmus in 40 cases by Fred Harbert, an otolaryngologist at Jefferson Medical College in Philadelphia. Just as Bárány reported in his 1921 paper, Harbert (1970) noted that: "In the typical reaction, the nystagmus is vertical when looking away from and rotary when looking toward the involved lowermost ear" (p. 299) (see Figure 11.3). The vertical component beat upward while the torsional component beat toward the lower ear. Based on the work of Janos Szentágothai (1950), the famous Hungarian anatomist who cannulated the membranous canals of cats to permit stimulation of an individual canal by increasing or decreasing the endolymphatic pressure (similar to Ewald's pneumatic hammer; see Figure 6.2), Harbert concluded that benign paroxysmal positional nystagmus had the typical features of nystagmus originating from the posterior semicircular canal. Szentágothai had shown that excitation of the posterior semicircular canal with ampullofugal endolymphatic flow produced contraction of the ipsilateral superior oblique and the contralateral inferior rectus

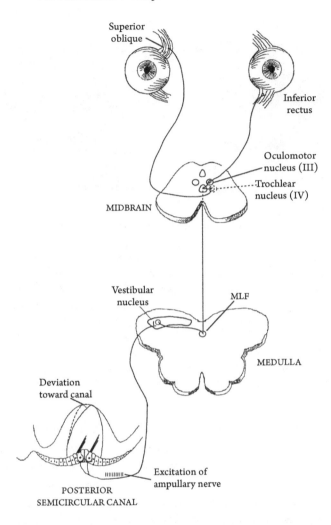

Figure 18.2 EXCITATORY CONNECTIONS FROM THE POSTERIOR SEMICIRCULAR CANAL TO THE VERTICAL EYE MUSCLES THAT RESULT IN A COMPENSATORY EYE MOVEMENT IN THE PLANE OF THAT CANAL. Excitation of the right posterior semicircular canal causes an activation of the right superior oblique and left inferior rectus, resulting in a torsional (clockwise) downward slow phase and torsional (counterclockwise) upward fast phase. MLF, medial longitudinal fasciculus.

muscles (Figure 18.2), whereas inhibition with ampullopetal endolymph flow resulted in relaxation of these muscles. Based on the pulling directions of the superior oblique and inferior rectus muscles (Figure 18.3), the changing rotary and vertical components of the nystagmus with changes in gaze direction originally described by Bárány were well explained.

In the example shown in Figure 18.2, excitation of the posterior semicircular canal afferent nerve on the right side primarily activates the right superior oblique

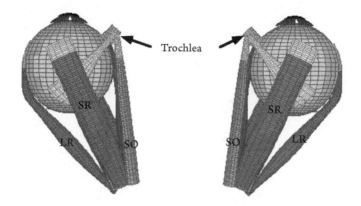

Figure 18.3 ANGLE OF INSERTION OF THE VERTICAL EYE MUSCLES LOOKING DOWN AT THE ORBITS. Note that the superior oblique (SO) tendon after going through the trochlea inserts in the back of the globe at approximately 60 degrees from straight ahead. With the eye turned inward, the SO is mainly a depressor of the globe; with the eye turned outward, the SO mainly produces torsion (rotation about an axis through the center of the pupil) of the globe. The inferior rectus (IR; not seen here) and superior rectus (SR) insert in the front of the globe approximately 30 degrees from the straight ahead. With the eye turned outward, the IR is a depressor of the globe; with the eye turned inward, the IR mainly produces torsion of the globe. The different angle of insertion of these vertical eye muscles explains the dysconjugate appearance of benign paroxysmal positional nystagmus. Source: Courtesy Joseph Demer MD, PhD, UCLA Ophthalmology.

and the left inferior rectus muscles, producing a vertical torsional eye movement with downward clockwise slow phase and upward counterclockwise fast phase. The upper pole of the eyes beat toward the ground in the head-hanging right position. Gaze to the right increases the torsional component and gaze to the left increases the vertical component as the eyes move away from and toward the main pulling direction of these vertical muscles, respectively. Another feature of the positional nystagmus predicted by the different angle of insertion of these eye muscles but not commented on by Bárány, Hallpike, or Schuknecht is that the induced nystagmus is dysconjugate with greater torsion in the undermost eye (the side with superior oblique activation—in this case, the right eye) in all gaze positions. This is a unique circumstance in that a single semicircular canal is activated by head movement, whereas with all normal physiologic head movements, a combination of canals on both sides are activated, producing conjugate eye movements.

The burst of activity originating from the posterior semicircular canal when the patient was placed in the critical position had to result in an ampullofugal (excitatory) deviation of the cupula in order to explain the direction of the vertical and torsional components of the observed nystagmus. In his 1969 paper on cupulolithiasis, Schuknecht quoted Harbert's findings and accepted his conclusion that the critical position change must result in an ampullofugal displacement of the cupula of the posterior semicircular canal, but he did not attempt to explain how such a displacement would result from a mass sitting on the utricular side of the cupula.

Problems with the Cupulolithiasis Theory

In 1973, Schuknecht published a second paper on cupulolithiasis in collaboration with Ralph Ruby. In this report, they described a third postmortem examination of a case with typical BPPV that showed a dense basophilic deposit on the cupula of the right posterior semicircular canal. They also reported results of their examination of 391 temporal bones from 245 individuals to determine the incidence of cupular deposits in temporal bone specimens from patients without a history of BPPV. Of the 391 specimens, small deposits were found in 125, medium deposits in 20, and large deposits comparable to the size found in the cupulolithiasis ears were found in 4. Deposits in the posterior semicircular canal were twice as common as those in the horizontal semicircular canal, whereas deposits in the superior semicircular canal were least frequent. The presence of the deposits bore no relationship to the state of preservation of the temporal bones, and the deposits were found as often in temporal bones judged to be normal as in those exhibiting pathological changes. They concluded that the cupular deposits of the size found in their 3 patients with the clinical syndrome of BPPV were uncommon in random temporal bone specimens and, therefore, were likely the cause of the clinical syndrome.

In their 1973 paper, Schuknecht and Ruby included a figure demonstrating the proposed mechanism of cupulolithiasis (as in Figure 17.2). As the posterior semicircular canal moves from an inferior to a superior position with relation to the utricle, the cupula is displaced in an ampullopetal direction. Schuknecht also used this figure in describing cupulolithiasis in the first edition of his textbook, *Pathology of the Ear*, published in 1974. In neither the 1973 paper nor his textbook did Schuknecht mention the discrepancy regarding the direction of cupular deviation noted in the 1969 and 1973 papers or in the paper by Harbert (1970) that concluded that the cupular deviation had to be ampullofugal (away from the utricle) to explain the typical nystagmus. This is surprising because in the 1969 paper, he had agreed that the nystagmus must result from ampullofugal displacement of the cupula of the posterior semicircular canal. Another problem raised in his 1973 paper was that in all three temporal bone specimens from patients with BPPV, the amorphous basophilic deposits seemed to be firmly attached to the cupula of the posterior semicircular canal, not likely easily dislodged. Thus, Schuknecht had to admit that the cupulolithiasis theory would not

explain the limited duration of the attack and the fatigability with repeated testing. In his earlier paper, he had explained these clinical features by suggesting that
the debris floats away from the cupula and becomes dispersed (see Figure 17.2).
The cupulolithiasis mechanism with an amorphous mass firmly attached to the
cupula would predict a sustained positional nystagmus for as long as the critical
position was maintained.

A key point that Schuknecht and the reviewers of the 1973 paper failed to
recognize is that the posterior semicircular canal is behind the utricle with a subject sitting erect and not in front of it as shown in Figure 17.2. If the position of
the posterior canal is reversed as it should be, the posterior canal is behind and
below the utricle when the subject is placed in the critical head-hanging position (Figure 18.4). A mass attached to the cupula would result in an ampullofugal (away from the utricle) displacement in the critical position as required
to explain the direction of the positional nystagmus. Schuknecht did finally

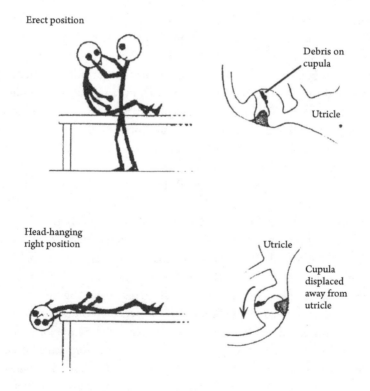

Figure 18.4 SCHUKNECHT'S CORRECTION OF THE INITIAL FIGURE, PLACING
THE UTRICLE IN THE PROPER POSITION SO THAT THE CUPULA WOULD
DEVIATE AWAY FROM THE UTRICLE IN THE STANDARD HEAD-HANGING
POSITION. Source: Reproduced with permission from Schuknecht HF. *Pathology of the Ear,* 2nd ed.
Philadelphia: Lea & Febiger, 1993.

recognize this error and made the appropriate changes in the second edition of his textbook, *Pathology of the Ear,* in 1993, but he still stuck with the cupulolithiasis theory even though it did not explain the brief duration of an attack and fatigability with repeated testing.

References

Dix MR, Hallpike CS. The pathology, symptomatology and diagnosis of certain common disorders of the vestibular system. *Proc R Soc Med* 1952;45:341–354.
Harbert F. Benign paroxysmal positional nystagmus. *Arch Ophthalmol* 1970;84:298–302.
Kiang NYS. HFS: A personal perspective. *Ann Otol Rhinol Laryngol (Suppl)* 1984;112:142–144.
Nadol JB. In memoriam: Harold F. Schuknecht, MD. *Am J Otol* 1997;18:135–136.
Schuknecht HF. Positional vertigo: Clinical and experimental observations. *Trans Am Acad Ophthalmol Otol* 1962:319–331.
Schuknecht HF. Cupulolithiasis. *Arch Otolaryngol* 1969;90:113–126.
Schuknecht HF. *Pathology of the Ear.* Cambridge, UK: Harvard University Press, 1974.
Schuknecht HF. *Pathology of the Ear,* 2nd ed. Philadelphia: Lea & Febiger, 1993.
Schuknecht HF, Ruby RRF. Cupulolithiasis. *Adv Oto-Rhino-Laryng* 1973;20:434–443.
Szentágothai J. The elementary vestibulo-ocular reflex. *J Neurophysiol* 1950;13:395–407.
Wittmaack K. Über Veränderungen im inneren Ohre nach Rotationen. *Verh Dtsch Ges Otol* 1909;18:150.
Wittmaack K. Kopfstellungsnystagmus [Comment]. *Acta Otolaryngol* 1927;11:156.

Schuknecht's Crusade Against Myths in Otology

Like Joseph Toynbee, Harold Schuknecht believed that the only way to develop rational treatments for inner ear diseases was to understand the pathology of these diseases. Quackery in otology did not disappear with the turn of the 20th century. Schuknecht (1992) noted,

> Regardless of how mysterious a disorder may be, most physicians feel obligated to counter with some form of medical or surgical treatment. The empirical approach to therapy is acceptable to many physicians, particularly if it can be based on an attractive, even unproven, concept of pathogenesis. The hypothetical explanation of disordered function can become widely accepted in spite of a serious lack of scientific support. When evidence emerges however that refutes the logic of a concept of pathogenesis, then that concept becomes a myth. No specialty in medicine, including neuro-otology, is immune to myths. (p. 124)

Surgical Treatments of Ménière's Disease

Schuknecht used his human temporal bone studies to "refute the conceptual validity of several popular otologic therapies." Probably the most controversial of these was the treatment of Ménière's disease with endolymphatic shunt surgery. In 1927, Stacey Guild, an anatomist at the University of Michigan, theorized that endolymph was formed in the labyrinth and flowed through the endolymphatic duct into the endolymphatic sac, where it was absorbed (see Figure 13.1A). Like cerebrospinal fluid, there was a continuous circulation of endolymph. After Hallpike and Cairns and Yamakawa demonstrated that endolymphatic hydrops was the main pathology associated with Ménière's disease (Figure 19.1), "otolaryngologists seized the gauntlet and attacked the endolymphatic sac with vigor

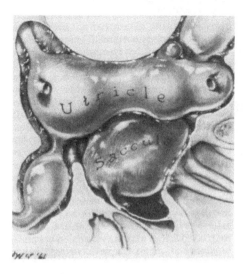

Figure 19.1 SCHUKNECHT'S DRAWING OF THE DILATED MEMBRANOUS
LABYRINTH IN MÉNIÈRE'S DISEASE. The drawing was made from a three-dimensional
model developed from serial microscopic sections of the inner ear of a patient with
Ménière's disease. Source: From Schuknecht HF. *Pathology of the Ear.* Cambridge, Harvard
University Press, 1974.

and enthusiasm" (Schuknecht, 1992, p. 125). Assuming there was a problem with
resorption of endolymph in the endolymphatic sac, a shunt of the endolymphatic
sac was an obvious remedy, analogous to shunting hydrocephalus in the brain.
Shunting the endolymphatic sac was technically difficult, however, considering
that the entire amount of endolymph is less than 1 ml. Furthermore, Schuknecht
argued "the concept that the endolymph sac can be drained to relieve endolymphatic hydrops is a pedantic notion at best" (p. 125). He had studied numerous human temporal bone specimens of patients who had had shunts placed in
the endolymphatic sac, and in every case the shunt devices were ensheathed in
fibrous tissue. Also in animal studies, shunts placed in the endolymphatic sac
could not be kept open for more than a few hours (Schuknecht, 1986).

Furthermore, Schuknecht argued that endolymph flow through the endolymphatic duct was either blocked or markedly diminished in most cases of
Ménière's disease, and often the endolymphatic sac was too small to accept any
kind of shunt device. A placebo-controlled study performed in Scandinavia by
Thomsen and colleagues (1981) supported Schuknecht's (1992) argument.
Unlike other therapies in medicine, placebo-controlled studies of surgical
techniques are rare. Thomsen and colleagues compared the outcome of three
groups of patients with classical Ménière's disease. One group was treated with
endolymphatic shunt surgery, a second group underwent mastoid surgery similar to the first but no shunting (placebo surgery), and the third group received

standard medical therapy without surgery. Follow-up during the next several years showed that both surgical groups did better than the medically treated group, but there was no significant difference between the two surgical groups. This study emphasized the important placebo effect of any type of surgery. In 1992, Schuknecht concluded that "the myth survives, and hundreds, possibly thousands, of endolymphatic shunt procedures are performed every year worldwide with benefits that are probably attributable to the placebo effect" (p. 126).

Viral Neurolabyrinthitis

Every year, more than 4000 people in the United States are stricken with "sudden deafness" usually involving just one side although rarely involving both sides. Traditionally, otologists considered sudden deafness to result from blockage of blood supply to the inner ear so that frequently patients were hospitalized for administration of anticoagulants, vasodilators, and blood viscosity reducing agents. Throughout the years, Schuknecht collected a total of 12 temporal bone specimens from patients who had experienced sudden unilateral deafness. None of these specimens showed abnormalities in the vascular systems. However, he found a selective degeneration in the organ of Corti, primarily involving the sensory cells. These changes were identical to those seen in specimens from patients with sudden hearing loss due to known viral diseases such as mumps and measles, and they were completely different from those seen in specimens in which there was known vascular occlusion. Schuknecht (1992) concluded that the vascular hypothesis was a myth for most cases of sudden deafness and that aggressive vascular therapies caused more harm than benefit.

Although some patients with sudden deafness also experience vertigo, most have hearing loss alone. This suggests that certain viruses have a preference for the sensory epithelium of the cochlea. The reciprocal of this notion is that other viruses have a predilection for the vestibular end organs. Annually in the United States, 4000–5000 patients have the sudden new onset of vertigo that gradually resolves over 1 or 2 weeks. This clinical syndrome, called vestibular neuronitis by Dix and Hallpike in their classic 1952 paper (see Chapter 16), was characterized by acute prolonged vertigo with normal hearing and otherwise normal neurologic function. Dix and Hallpike concluded that it resulted from "some form of organic disease confined to the vestibular apparatus and localized, in all probability, to its peripheral nervous pathways up to and including the vestibular nuclei in the brainstem" (p. 343). They called the condition vestibular neuronitis because they believed that this was "a term comprehensive enough to encompass this uncertainty" (p. 343). On studying the temporal bones of numerous patients with vestibular neuronitis, Schuknecht noted a consistent pattern of atrophy of

vestibular nerve branches and of the vestibular sensory epithelium (Figure 19.2).
Again, these changes were identical to those associated with known viral inner ear
syndromes, such as herpes zoster infection of the vestibular system. He therefore
coined the term "vestibular neuritis" referring to a discrete degenerative neuropa-
thy of the vestibular nerve trunks (Schuknecht and Kitamura, 1981). There was
no evidence of vascular disease in any of his specimens, and he noted that the
selective atrophy was not consistent with a vascular mechanism.

There was also strong epidemiological evidence that the syndromes of sudden deafness and vestibular neuritis were caused by viral infection of the inner
ear (Schuknecht, 1985a). Approximately 50% of such patients report an upper
respiratory tract illness or a flu-like illness at approximately the time of onset
of the inner ear symptoms. Both syndromes occur in epidemics, may affect

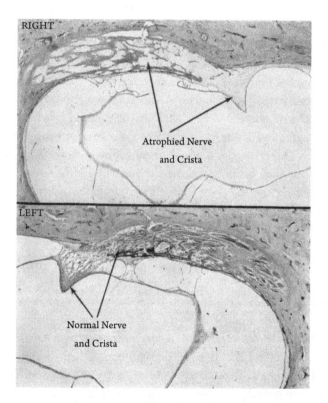

Figure 19.2 VESTIBULAR NEURITIS FROM SCHUKNECHT'S TEMPORAL
BONE BANK. Histological cross section of the horizontal semicircular canal ampulla
showing severe atrophy of the vestibular nerve and the crista (sensory epithelium)
in the right ear and normal nerve and crista in the left ear. The cupula is not seen due
to postmortem shrinkage. At age 85 years, this woman had acute onset of vertigo,
nausea, and vomiting that gradually resolved over weeks. She had normal hearing but
absent response to caloric stimulation on the right side. She died of unrelated causes
2 years later. Source: Courtesy Harold Schuknecht (1979).

several members of the same family, and erupt more commonly in the spring and early summer. The diagnosis of a specific viral infection in a given patient is more difficult, however. Antibody studies can demonstrate that a virus infected the patient but do not prove that the infectious agent caused the inner ear damage. Furthermore, isolation of an infectious agent from the throat or other tissue other than the inner ear does not prove a causal relationship between the virus and the inner ear disease. Although a few viruses have been cultured directly from perilymph samples in infected ears, this is not a practical method for routine diagnosis of viral infections of the inner ear. Recent studies suggest that many cases of vestibular neuritis result from activation of a latent herpes simplex virus that lies dormant in the vestibular nerve ganglia (Scarpa's ganglia).

In his later years, Schuknecht (1985a) coined the term "neurolabyrinthitis" to cover the spectrum of viral inner ear disorders. He argued that viruses selectively involve the vestibular and cochlear nerves and their branches and any of the sensory receptors so that any combination of vestibular and auditory symptoms is possible. Certain viruses seem to be selective for the vestibular and/or cochlear part of the inner ear, but many affect both parts. He believed that because viral labyrinthitis and viral neuritis could not be separated on clinical grounds and often there was some combination of nerve and end organ involvement, neurolabyrinthitis was a more practical clinical term.

Based on his later experience of temporal bone studies in patients with viral inner ear syndromes, Schuknecht reassessed his interpretation of the patients with benign paroxysmal positional vertigo (BPPV) reported by Lindsay and Hemenway in 1956 (see Chapter 17). These cases that Schuknecht initially ascribed to occlusion of the anterior vestibular artery provided the impetus for his theory of cupulolithiasis. On reviewing the temporal bone specimens of Lindsay and Hemenway and Hallpike and colleagues, Schuknecht concluded that the pathology was most likely secondary to a viral rather than a vascular etiology (see Chapter 18). Schuknecht could find no evidence of vascular occlusion, and the atrophy of the vestibular nerve terminals and vestibular end organs reminded him of the changes seen with viral neurolabyrinthitis in other patients. A remarkable feature in these cases that Schuknecht did not address is the selective involvement of the superior part of the vestibular labyrinth with sparing of the inferior part. This indeed was the feature that initially led Schuknecht to speculate on occlusion of the anterior vestibular artery and that because the posterior semicircular canal was the only canal spared, it must be the source of BPPV. This dichotomy between involvement of the superior and inferior part of the vestibular labyrinth has been consistently seen in patients with the clinical syndrome of vestibular neuritis or neurolabyrinthitis. If the syndrome is indeed secondary to a viral infection, then the virus or viruses must have a predilection for the superior part of the vestibular labyrinth. Possibly, the latent herpes simplex virus has a predilection for the ganglia of the superior branch of the vestibular nerve.

Like Ménière, Schuknecht tried to save patients from needless and potentially dangerous treatments. When he was asked to recommend the best treatment among the many treatments that have been recommended for these presumed viral inner ear disorders, Schuknecht (1985b) commented that

> there is no treatment I'm aware of. Certainly vasodilators, antibiotics, probably steroids—none of these drugs are really effective drugs for the treatment of viral disorders, as you all know. So all I'm making a plea for is a more logical approach to these disorders and for us not to be carried away by some therapeutic concept that's being imposed upon us by well-meaning colleagues, maybe pharmaceutical houses, and others. (p. 13)

Questionable Surgical Procedures

Schuknecht was a tireless crusader against surgical procedures that he considered to have little scientific underpinning yet provided significant risk to the patient (e.g., endolymphatic shunt surgery mentioned previously). Two popular surgeries that he considered in that category were vascular loop surgery and perilymph fistula surgery. Several surgeons suggested that compression of the auditory and vestibular nerve trunks by vascular loops of normal arteries was a common cause of hearing loss, tinnitus, and vertigo, and even possibly Ménière's disease. An article titled "Disabling Positional Vertigo," published in the *New England Journal of Medicine* in 1984, spawned a flurry of interest in vascular decompression surgery by both neurosurgeons and otologists (Janetta et al., 1984). Dramatic improvement was reported in patients with "disabling positional vertigo" after surgically removing vascular loops that were compressing the eighth cranial nerve. The problem was that the clinical syndrome was ill-defined, and there were no diagnostic tests that could confirm the condition prior to surgical exploration of the brain. A few of the patients in the *New England Journal* paper had typical symptoms of BPPV. Reisser and Schuknecht (1991) noted that vascular loops are common in normal subjects without symptoms. On reviewing Schuknecht's temporal bone specimens, they found that such loops were in the internal auditory canal in 12.3% of 1327 temporal bones. Of these, 5 had unexplained unilateral hearing loss, but in 3 of them the loops were located in the opposite ears and 2 had the loops in both ears. Two of the cases with vascular loops had unexplained tinnitus, but one was in the uninvolved ear. They concluded that there were no clinical manifestations that could be attributed to vascular loops in the internal auditory canal and that his temporal bone observations seriously challenged the concept that arterial loops anywhere along the course of the auditory and vestibular nerve trunks were the cause of auditory–vestibular disorders: "The practice of performing a suboccipital craniotomy for the purpose of cushioning these nerve trunks against the pulsation of arteries does not seem reasonable in view of these findings" (Schuknecht, 1992, p. 125).

Traumatic rupture of the inner ear membranes produces a perilymph leak called a perilymph fistula. Some otologists have suggested that spontaneous perilymph fistulae are a common cause of hearing loss, tinnitus, and vertigo. Schuknecht had done extensive work on trauma to the inner ear in animals, and he was highly skeptical of this concept of a spontaneous perilymph fistula. He was particularly struck by the fact that when he intentionally ruptured the membranous labyrinth when performing a cochleosacculotomy operation for Ménière's syndrome (a procedure in which a fistula is intentionally made in the labyrinth to relieve the internal pressure), patients rarely had auditory or vestibular symptoms as a result, with less than 25% showing evidence of postoperative sensorineural hearing loss. Also, the perilymphatic space is routinely entered during stapedectomy surgery for otosclerosis, whereas postoperative auditory or vestibular symptoms are unusual. Some otologists, however, were performing several hundred explorations of the middle ear for perilymph fistulae every year. Schuknecht (1992) concluded that "perilymph fistula is a proven reality following several different types of stress-related incidents. However, the idea that it is a common cause of audiovestibular symptoms that are not related to a stressful incident is a myth" (p. 126).

The Final Years

Harold Schuknecht's scholarly productivity included more than 300 original articles, editorials, and reviews and seven books on the anatomy, pathology and surgery of the ear. His temporal bone collection at the Massachusetts Eye and Ear Infirmary contained more than 1500 sets of clinically well-documented specimens. Without a doubt, his most lasting contribution is his textbook, *Pathology of the Ear*, the second edition of which was completed in 1993 just 4 years before his death. Schuknecht began the second edition of his text with a quote from Joseph Toynbee:

> If we carefully survey the history of the rise and progress of aural [surgery] as a distinct branch of scientific surgery one main cause of the disrepute into which it has fallen may be traced to the neglect of the pathology of the organ of hearing.

Throughout his career, Schuknecht demonstrated a burning desire to understand the pathophysiology of disease processes. As Chairman of the Department
of Otology and Laryngology at the Harvard Medical School and Chief of
Otolaryngology at Massachusetts Eye and Ear Infirmary from 1960 to 1987,
Schuknecht was responsible for training many of the now chairmen of departments of otolaryngology worldwide. After retiring from his administrative and
clinical activities in 1987, he continued to teach and conduct research, focusing
on his temporal bone collection and the second edition of his textbook.

In 1996, while he was attending a medical meeting in Vancouver, Canada,
Schuknecht had several recurrent spells of right-sided weakness typical of
transient ischemia attacks. He had had an episode of transient aphasia approximately 5 years previously, but otherwise there had been no prior warnings.
He flew back to Boston and although his physician wanted him to immediately go to the emergency room, he preferred to stay at home overnight and
enter the hospital the next day. He had his wife Anne make freshly baked corn-
bread smothered with milk and sugar. Since he was a child in South Dakota,
this was his favorite meal or snack. He reminded Anne that he wanted to be
cremated because he still had disturbing memories of his mother's funeral
and the several days that she was laid out for viewing. Despite his strict religious upbringing, he had lost interest in religion once he had left the farm
and started college. He had a peaceful night without any further spells, and
the next day he entered Massachusetts General Hospital to undergo a carotid
endarterectomy (a procedure to remove plaque from the blocked artery).
One complication after another followed so that he was not able to leave the
intensive care unit for the next 6½ weeks. After a quadruple coronary bypass
operation, he had a massive stroke, leaving him paralyzed and unable to com-
municate. Day after day, he sat in a chair in the intensive care unit watching
the activities going on around him but unable to respond. His wife knew that
he wanted out of the situation, and finally she was able to arrange for him to
leave the intensive care unit and enter a hospice, where he died peacefully
within a day (Anne Schuknecht, personal communication, 1998).

References

Dix MR, Hallpike CS. The pathology, symptomatology and diagnosis of certain common disor-
    ders of the vestibular system. *Proc R Soc Med* 1952;45:341-354.
Guild SR. The circulation of the endolymph. *Am J Anat* 1927;39:57–81.
Janetta PJ, Moller MB, Moller ARC. Disabling positional vertigo. *N Engl J Med* 1984;
    310:1700–1705.
Lindsay JR, Hemenway WG. Postural vertigo due to unilateral sudden partial loss of vestibular
    function. *Ann Otol Rhinol Laryngol* 1956;65:692–706.

Reisser C, Schuknecht HF. The anterior inferior cerebellar artery in the internal auditory canal. *Laryngoscope* 1991;101:761–766.

Schuknecht HF. Neurolabyrinthitis: Viral infections of the peripheral auditory and vestibular systems. In *Hearing Loss and Dizziness.* Nomura Y, ed. Tokyo: Igaku-Shoin, 1985a, pp 1–12.

Schuknecht HF. Neurolabyrinthitis: Questions and answers. In *Hearing Loss and Dizziness.* Nomura Y, ed. Tokyo: Igaku-Shoin, 1985b, pp 13–15.

Schuknecht HF. Endolymphatic hydrops: Can it be controlled? *Ann Otol Rhinol Laryngol* 1986;95:36–39.

Schuknecht HF. Myths in neurotology. *Am J Otol* 1992;13:124–126.

Schuknecht HF. *Pathology of the Ear,* 2nd ed. Philadelphia: Lea & Febiger, 1993.

Schuknecht HF, Kitamura K. Vestibular neuritis: Second Louis H. Clerf lecture. *Ann Otol Rhinol Laryngol* 1981;90(1, Pt 2):1–19.

Thomsen J, Brettan P, Tos M, et al. Placebo effect of surgery for Meniere's disease. *Arch Otolaryngol* 1981;107:271.

SECTION 6

THE PIECES OF THE PUZZLE COME TOGETHER

By the late 20th century, all the pieces of the puzzle were in place for the development of a simple cure for benign paroxysmal positional vertigo (BPPV). Harold Schuknecht had focused attention on the posterior semicircular canal with his cupulolithiasis model, and Joe McClure had clarified the difference between cupulolithiasis and canalithiasis. Two clinicians—Alain Semont, a physical therapist in Paris, and John Epley, an otolaryngologist in Oregon—pioneered the development of the treatment maneuvers. Both faced broad skepticism from the medical community regarding their claims of cures for BPPV, and both doggedly persisted with treatment trials despite the skepticism. The treatment maneuvers have subsequently evolved based on experience in large treatment trials and on improved understanding of the underlying mechanism of different variants of BPPV.

Semont and Epley Maneuvers

Until 1980, treatment of benign paroxysmal positional vertigo (BPPV) mainly consisted of reassuring patients of the benign nature of the condition along with a recommendation that they avoid the critical position changes that induced the vertigo. Most patients had a spontaneous remission, although not infrequently the condition recurred. The same benign course was seen whether BPPV occurred after head trauma or an ear infection or if it occurred spontaneously. Although brain lesions could produce positional vertigo and nystagmus, the stereotyped torsional vertical nystagmus of BPPV was a reliable signature of a benign inner ear disorder.

Treatments Based on the Cupulolithiasis Theory

In 1974, Richard Gacek, an otologic surgeon in Rochester, New York, reported that BPPV could be cured by selectively sectioning the ampullary nerve from the posterior semicircular canal. The procedure was performed under a local anesthetic, and the BPPV disappeared immediately after the nerve was sectioned. This provided unequivocal evidence that BPPV was originating from the posterior semicircular canal. However, the surgical procedure was not without risk (approximately 1 in 10 lost hearing), so it was considered only for patients with severe incapacitating symptoms.

In the late 1970s, two neurologists, Thomas Brandt from Germany and Robert Daroff from the United States, introduced a physical therapy approach for treatment of BPPV (Brandt and Daroff, 1980). Instead of recommending that patients avoid the critical position that induced BPPV, they had patients perform positional exercises that repeatedly induced BPPV. Based on Schuknecht's cupulolithiasis theory, they believed that the physical therapy "provided a mechanical means to promote loosening and ultimate dispersion of the otolithic debris from the cupula" (p. 485). They had their patients sit on the edge of a bed and then fall to one side, triggering the typical attack of BPPV (Figure 20.1). Patients

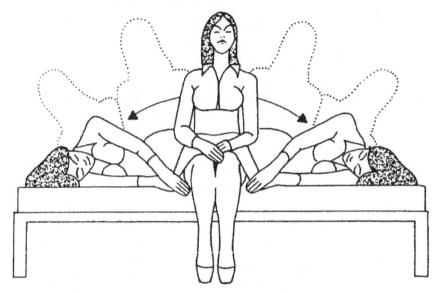

Figure 20.1 POSITIONAL EXERCISES DEVELOPED BY BRANDT AND DAROFF.
Source: Reproduced with permission from Brandt T, Daroff RB. Physical therapy for benign paroxysmal positional vertigo. *Arch Otolaryngol* 1980;106:484–485.

remained in this position until the evoked vertigo disappeared, and then they returned to the sitting position for approximately 30 seconds before assuming the opposite head-down position for another 30 seconds. Typically, vertigo was induced only on one side, but patients alternated between sides, always stopping in the sitting erect position in between. The sequence of positionings during each session was repeated until the vertigo subsided (fatigued). Patients were instructed to perform these positional exercises every 3 hours while awake until they had 2 consecutive vertigo-free days. Some patients were hospitalized for several weeks undergoing repeated exercises.

In 1980, Brandt and Daroff reported that 66 of 67 patients were cured of their BPPV after performing these positional exercises for 3–14 days, with most requiring 7–10 days. Of interest, they noted that approximately one-third of patients reported a spontaneous abrupt disappearance of symptoms during the course of treatment. Only 2 of the 66 patients experienced a recurrence of BPPV after several months, and each of these again responded to a course of the physical therapy. They argued that the fatigability of BPPV during individual sessions and the abrupt termination of BPPV in approximately one-third of the patients argued against a central nervous system habituation and in favor of their mechanical hypothesis (i.e., dispersion of otolith debris from the cupula). Their physical therapy program offered the first possibility for a simple cure of BPPV, but many patients refused to repeatedly induce the distressing vertigo, particularly those who developed severe nausea and vomiting.

Semont's Maneuver

In the 1980s, a physical therapist in Paris, Alain Semont, described a physical therapy maneuver (the "liberatory maneuver") that he found highly effective in curing BPPV after a single treatment. Like the Brandt–Daroff exercises, Semont's maneuver was initially designed to dislodge debris attached to the cupula of the posterior semicircular canal. With the maneuver, he positioned patents into the critical position that induced BPPV, similar to the start of the Brandt–Daroff exercises. However, instead of returning to the sitting upright position, the patient was thrown across to the opposite head-down position with a rapid thrust. Semont briefly mentioned the dramatic cures of BPPV with his maneuver in a paper on vestibular rehabilitation published with J. M. Sterkers in 1980. Semont visited the author's clinic at UCLA in the early 1980s and demonstrated the maneuver, but the faculty were skeptical of the benefit because it seemed to be just a variation of the Brandt–Daroff exercises without a clear theoretical basis for how it worked.

In 1988, Semont, along with colleagues Freyss and Vitte, reported the results of performing the maneuver on 711 patients during an 8-year period. They described the maneuver as follows:

> The patient is laid on the ipsilateral side to the sick ear with his head slightly declined. The nystagmus can appear: In this condition one must wait until it stops. If nothing happens, the head is turned 45° facing up in order to have the cupula in the perpendicular plane to gravity. In this position, after a variable latency, the paroxysmal rotatory nystagmus rolling toward the examination table appears. One waits until it has completely stopped and then the patient is left in this position for 2 or 3 minutes. Then, holding the patient's head and neck with two hands, he is swung quickly to the opposite side. The speed of the head must be zero at the very moment the head touches the examination table. Then a rotatory nystagmus appears still rolling toward the sick ear which is now the higher one. It must not be an inverted nystagmus. The nystagmus is slightly different: wide amplitude, slower frequency, not so paroxysmal as the original one. If nothing happens the head is slowly turned nearly to 90° facing up and then quickly turned to 45° facing down. Then the nystagmus occurs. The patient must stay in this last position for at least 5 minutes and is brought back to orthostatism very, very slowly. (p. 291)

Semont and colleagues (1988) reported that more than 84% of the patients were cured after a single maneuver and 93% after two maneuvers. They reported a recurrence rate of 4%. They went on to state that other European physicians, including physicians in Switzerland, Italy, and Belgium, who were taught the maneuver found a similar cure rate. They concluded that "the results confirm the hypothesis of the cupula being modified in its density, but cannot discriminate between cupulolithiasis and floating substances" (p. 292). This report was widely discussed, but skepticism abounded. No doubt the complicated description of the maneuver and the lack of a clear explanation of what it was designed to do limited its acceptance.

Cupulolithiasis Versus Canalithiasis

Although the cupulolithiasis theory of Schuknecht had gained general acceptance, there were two important features of BPPV not adequately explained: the transient duration of the nystagmus and the fatigability with repeated positioning. In his original 1962 paper, Schuknecht suggested that the otoconial debris might dislodge from the cupula and float away, allowing the cupula to return to its normal position, and that the particles might become dispersed within the endolymph with repeated positioning (see Figure 17.2). However, when his subsequent postmortem studies showed that the otolithic debris was firmly attached to the cupula of the posterior semicircular canal, these possibilities seemed less likely. One would expect that a mass firmly attached to the cupula would result in a persistent deviation of the cupula and persistent vertigo and nystagmus as long as the critical position was maintained. Central adaptation phenomena might eventually suppress the nystagmus and vertigo, but this process would require many minutes to hours, not the seconds' duration of typical BPPV.

In the late 1970s, Joseph McClure, a Canadian physician with a background in mechanical engineering, recognized these problems with the cupulolithiasis theory and began to experiment with mechanical models of the inner ear to determine if these issues could be resolved (Joseph McClure, personal communication, 1998). His simple model consisted of a water bottle representing the utricular chamber and two attached rounded tubes representing the posterior and anterior semicircular canals (Figure 20.2). He placed mercury in the bottle to represent the otoconial debris and noted that repeated positional changes from the sitting to head-hanging position caused the mercury to enter the posterior semicircular canal, becoming trapped on the canal side of the cupula. McClure recognized that freely floating debris in this location could readily explain both the paroxysmal nature of BPPV and fatigability. When the subject moved from a sitting to head-hanging position, the debris would move away from the cupula, causing the necessary ampullofugal flow and then coming to rest at the most

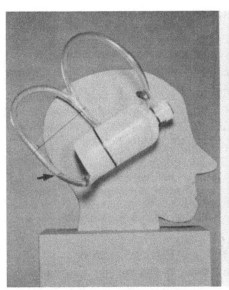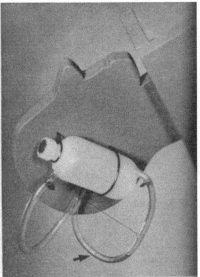

Figure 20.2 McClure's model of the inner ear illustrating free-
floating debris (mercury) in the posterior semicircular canal.
The water bottle represents the utricle, and the circular tubes represent the posterior
and anterior semicircular canals. (Left) With the subject sitting up, the mercury
(arrow) lies at the bottom of the posterior canal next to the cupula. (Right) With the
head back, the mercury moves away from the cupula (arrow), causing the cupula to
deviate away from the utricle, which in turn causes an excitatory stimulation of the
afferent nerve. Source: Reproduced with permission from Hall SF, Ruby RRF, McClure JA. The
mechanics of benign paroxysmal vertigo. *J Otolaryngol* 1979;8:151–158.

inferior position in the posterior semicircular canal. With repeated positioning,
the debris could become dispersed, accounting for fatigability.

S. F. Hall was a resident in otolaryngology at the University of Western Ontario
when he became interested in McClure's model as part of his research rotation.
Hall presented the model and its predictions at the 32nd annual meeting of the
Canadian Otolaryngological Society in Quebec in 1978, and along with men-
tors Ralph Ruby and Joe McClure, he published a paper describing the model in
1979. In the paper, Hall, Ruby, and McClure suggested that BPPV might be sub-
classified into two types: fatigable and nonfatigable. Nonfatigable BPPV was due
to cupulolithiasis as described by Schuknecht, whereas fatigable BPPV resulted
from freely moving debris within the posterior semicircular canal as illustrated in
McClure's model (canalithiasis—"stones in the canal"). They argued,

> It is easy to imagine that with repeated changes in head position, some
> of the free floating statoconia could become trapped within another
> part of the labyrinth. With fewer and fewer particles in motion, less cur-
> rent would be created and fatigue would be observed. (p. 153)

206 SECTION 6. THE PIECES OF THE PUZZLE COME TOGETHER

They described a simple way for bringing back BPPV after it had been fatigued. They had the patient sit with the head well down between the knees with the neck flexed for 3–5 minutes; invariably, the positional vertigo would be present on repeat positioning. They said little about treatment of BPPV in their paper other than to suggest that surgery might be appropriate for cupulolithiasis but not for canalithiasis. When later asked if he had tried any maneuvers to treat patients with BPPV based on his canalithiasis model, McClure indicated that he had tried positioning a few patients but the results were equivocal and he did not persist with the treatment maneuvers.

Epley's Maneuver

When John Epley finished his otolaryngology training at Stanford in 1965, he returned to his hometown of Portland, Oregon, and entered private practice, focusing mainly on ear surgery (John Epley, personal communication, 1998). He saw numerous cases of BPPV and performed the Gacek singular neurectomy surgery on several intractable cases (cutting the ampullary nerve from the posterior canal). Although patients often described other types of dizziness in addition to the typical vertigo attacks, all of these symptoms were cured after singular neurectomy. For example, some patients with BPPV had brief sensations of spinning or rolling while jogging or riding horseback, whereas others noted brief spinning sensations when accelerating or decelerating in an automobile. In a paper published in 1980, he described these additional symptoms and suggested that they probably resulted from the same mechanism that triggers positional vertigo (i.e., movement of the particles within the posterior semicircular canal). Epley did not distinguish between cupulolithiasis and canalithiasis but, rather, suggested that debris was both attached to the cupula and free floating in most cases of BPPV. However, he recognized that debris moving within the narrow semicircular canal would be much more effective in deviating the cupula than an equal amount of debris floating within the ampulla next to the cupula. He saw the analogy of the bolus of particles acting as a piston moving within the narrow confines of the semicircular canal that, according to Pascal's formula, would lead to increased force acting on the cupula. If this bolus of debris could move so easily with position change, it should be possible to move it around and out of the posterior semicircular canal and into the utricle with appropriate positional changes.

After experimenting with several positional maneuvers, by 1980 Epley convinced himself that he could cure most cases of BPPV with a simple maneuver that rotated the patient around the plane of the posterior semicircular canal with the head back in the head-hanging position. It took another 10 years, however, before he was able to convince other people of his simple cure for

BPPV. Early on, he learned that patients were subject to recurrence of BPPV, particularly in the first few days after the maneuver was performed. He recalled performing the maneuver successfully on a farmer who came to Oregon from Idaho in the early 1980s. The farmer called him a few days later, however, saying that the positional vertigo recurred when he crawled under his porch to chase out an animal that had taken up residence there (John Epley, personal communication, 1998). After this, Epley recommended that his patients stay upright as much as possible for at least 2 days after the procedure was performed. With these new instructions, he believed that he achieved a better cure rate. He gathered together all of his experience in treating BPPV with his particle repositioning maneuver and sent a paper to the *American Journal of Otology* in 1985. After not hearing from the editor for approximately 1 year, Epley wrote to the journal and finally received a letter of apology stating that they had forgotten to mail him his letter of rejection. The reviewer of the paper concluded "his findings were not consistent with existing theory" (John Epley, personal communication, 1998).

Epley also described his maneuver at several meetings and at courses presented at the American Academy of Otolaryngology. Skepticism abounded, and few were convinced of his claims. He recalled that during one of his presentations at an Academy course, one of the participants stood up in the middle of his presentation and angrily walked out (John Epley, personal communication, 1998). In his critique of the course, the angry participant indicated "he had more important things to do with his time than listen to someone's pet theories." With the publication of the physical therapy maneuver for treating BPPV by Semont and colleagues in 1988, renewed interest began to develop for a simple cure for BPPV. In October 1991, Epley sent a paper to *Otolaryngology Head and Neck Surgery* describing the results of his maneuver on 30 patients with BPPV treated between January 1, 1988, and July 1, 1990. After two revisions, the paper was finally accepted on March 1992. Epley reported that all 30 patients were cured with his maneuver, and he concluded that the maneuver was simpler and more effective than any other treatment modality for BPPV. Typically, he premedicated the patients either with transdermal scopolamine the night before or with diazepam given orally 1 hour before the maneuver. He used a five-position cycle designed to rotate the particles around and out of the involved semicircular canal (Figure 20.3). He also used a vibrator attached to the mastoid on the affected side, which he believed helped mobilize particles that may be adherent to the cupula or membranous labyrinth. After completing the maneuver, patients were advised to keep their heads relatively upright for 48 hours so that the loose debris would not gravitate back into the posterior semicircular canal. He noted that 30% of the patients experienced one or more recurrences of BPPV, but each responded well to retreatment with the maneuver.

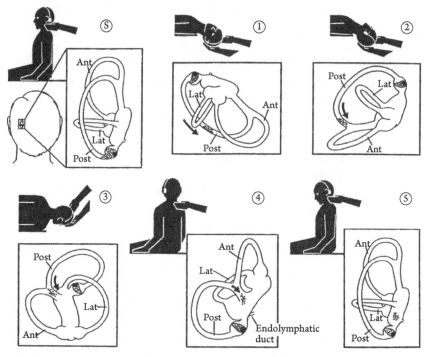

Figure 20.3 EPLY'S POSITIONAL MANEUVER DESIGNED TO REMOVE DEBRIS
FROM THE POSTERIOR SEMICIRCULAR CANAL. In the sitting position (S), the clot
of calcium carbonate crystals lies at the bottom-most position within the posterior
canal. Movement to the head-hanging position (1) causes the clot to move away from
the cupula, producing an excitatory burst of activity in the ampullary nerve from the
posterior canal (ampullofugal displacement of the cupula). Each subsequent position
change causes the clot to move further around the canal and finally into the utricle (as
shown in 4 and 5). Source: Reproduced with permission from Epley JM. The canalith repositioning
procedure: For treatment of benign paroxysmal positional vertigo. *Otolaryngol Head Neck Surg*
1992;107:399–404.

Visualization of the Free-Floating Otolith Debris

Despite the excellent results for the particle repositioning maneuver reported
by Epley, the treatment was still not generally accepted. During this same time,
Lorne Parnes, an otologic surgeon, began working with Joe McClure at the
University of Western Ontario to develop a better surgical treatment for BPPV.
McClure had shown that the posterior semicircular canal could be effectively
blocked in animals by drilling into its bony wall and inserting a plug of ground-
up bone and glue. Parnes adapted the operation for patients with BPPV and
found that just as with Gacek's singular neurectomy, patients with BPPV had
a dramatic cure after the posterior semicircular canal was blocked (Parnes and

McClure, 1990). In the process of performing the operation with a surgical microscope, Parnes removed a small piece of bone from the bony wall of the posterior semicircular canal prior to inserting the bone plug and noted freely floating white chalky particles in the endolymph of the posterior semicircular canal (Parnes and McClure, 1992). The particles were in the exact location predicted by McClure's canalithiasis model and Epley's maneuver. When Parnes showed a video of these freely moving particles at a national meeting, everyone began jumping on the canalithiasis bandwagon. Suddenly, Epley's maneuver did not seem so far-fetched. Seeing the particles was believing. Many physicians began using the treatment, and numerous articles were published confirming its effectiveness.

References

Brandt T, Daroff RB. Physical therapy for benign paroxysmal positional vertigo. *Arch Otolaryngol* 1980;106:484–485.

Epley JM. New dimensions of benign paroxysmal positional vertigo. *Otolaryngol Head Neck Surg* 1980;88:599–605.

Epley JM. The canalith repositioning procedure: For treatment of benign paroxysmal positional vertigo. *Otolaryngol Head Neck Surg* 1992;107:399–404.

Gacek R. Transection of the posterior ampullary nerve for the relief of benign paroxysmal positional vertigo. *Ann Otol Rhinol Laryngol* 1974;83:596–605.

Hall SF, Ruby RRF, McClure JA. The mechanics of benign paroxysmal vertigo. *J Otolaryngol* 1979;8:151–158.

Parnes LS, McClure JA. Posterior semicircular canal occlusion for intractable benign positional vertigo. *Ann Otol Rhinol Laryngol* 1990;99:330–333.

Schuknecht HF. Positional vertigo: Clinical and experimental observations. *Trans Am Acad Ophthalmol Otol* 1962:319–331.

Semont A, Sterkers JM. Rééducation vestibulaire. *Cah ORL* 1980;15:305–309.

Semont A, Freyss G, Vitte E. Curing the BPPV with a liberatory maneuver. *Adv Oto-Rhino-Laryng* 1988;42:290–293.

Evolution of Treatment Maneuvers for Benign Paroxysmal Positional Vertigo

Epley's Maneuver

Near the turn of the 21st century, as more physicians began performing the Epley maneuver for treatment of benign paroxysmal positional vertigo (BPPV), it became apparent that the procedure could be done at the time of the initial examination without the need for sedation or vibration. Furthermore, a modified version of the maneuver evolved that was more effective and easier to perform. Rather than the five positions of the original maneuver, just three are necessary for a good result. In the initial sitting position ("S" in Figure 20.3), the patient's head is turned 45 degrees toward the affected side, placing the posterior semicircular canal on that side in the sagittal plane (nasal–occipital plane). Moving the head back into the head-hanging position (position 1 in Figure 20.3) in the plane of the posterior canal on that side moves the debris halfway around the canal toward the utricle. The patient is then rolled across from position 1 to position 3 (not stopping at position 2), moving the debris further around the canal toward the utricle. By rolling across in one continuous movement, the debris moves more effectively due to the sustained acceleration of the single continuous movement. Positions 1 and 3 are held for approximately 30 seconds. The patient is then returned to the sitting position with head straight ahead (position 5), and the debris falls into the utricle if it has not already entered the utricle in position 3.

Although the majority of patients are cured after a single repositioning maneuver, the cure rate is improved by repeating the procedure until no vertigo or nystagmus occurs in any position. Occasionally, a patient will develop severe nausea and have to be rescheduled and premedicated with a vestibular suppressant drug. Also occasionally, vibration applied to the skull is useful if, rather than a burst of nystagmus with position change, the patient develops a slow persistent nystagmus suggesting that the otolith debris is stuck to the wall of the semicircular canal and not freely moving. A reliable sign that the repositioning maneuver is going to be successful is the production of a second identical burst of positional nystagmus when the patient is moved from the initial head-hanging position across to the opposite head-down position. This indicates that the particles are moving along in the canal in the correct direction toward the utricle. If, on the other hand, a burst of nystagmus in the reverse direction occurs when moving from one head-down position to the other, the particles are most likely moving in the wrong direction back toward the cupula, a sign that the repositioning maneuver will be unsuccessful. When this occurs, the patient most likely elevated the head during the movement from one head-down position to the other so the particles moved back in the opposite direction due to gravity. It is critical that the head stays down during this phase of the maneuver. When returning to the sitting position, at the end of the maneuver, patients may have a brief but violent burst of vertigo as late as 1 or 2 minutes after assuming the position. This delayed vertigo in the sitting position presumably occurs as the bolus of otolithic debris drops out of the common crus of the posterior and anterior semicircular canals into the utricle (as shown in Figure 20.3, position 4). Rarely, patients will develop a persistent vertigo and nystagmus immediately after returning to the sitting position. Epley (1995) speculated that this phenomenon resulted from jamming of the otolith debris (a "canalith jam") when migrating from a wider to a narrower segment, such as from the ampulla to the canal, or at the bifurcation of the common crus of the posterior and anterior canals. Repeating the particle repositioning maneuver with vibration applied to the skull will usually break up the canalith jam and cure the BPPV.

Semont's Maneuver

As noted previously, Semont's maneuver was initially designed based on the culpulolithiasis model of BPPV, essentially a variation of the Brandt–Daroff exercises to dislodge debris attached to the cupula. However, a modified version of the Semont maneuver evolved as the canalithiasis model became the accepted model of BPPV (Figure 21.1). For treating right-sided BPPV with the modified Semont maneuver, the patient turns the head 45 degrees toward the normal left side while sitting (position 1), placing the posterior semicircular canal on the right in the frontal plane (interaural plane). The patient then moves from the sitting position to the right lateral position in the plane of the right posterior canal, causing the debris to move halfway around the canal toward the utricle (position 2). The patient is then moved across to the opposite lateral position in the plane of the right posterior canal, causing the debris to roll further around the canal into the utricle. Both lateral positions are held for approximately 1 minute.

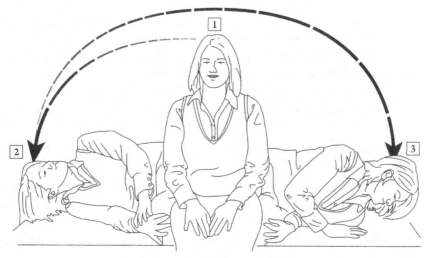

Figure 21.1 MODIFIED SEYMONT MANEUVER FOR TREATING RIGHT-
SIDED BPPV. (1) The patient is sitting facing forward and then turns the head 45
degrees to the left, placing the right posterior canal in the frontal plane. The patient is
then moved to the right lateral position (2) with the head remaining 45 degrees to the
left. This position is held for 2 minutes, and then the patient is taken all the way across
to the left lateral position (3) without stopping in the sitting position or changing head
position. After 2 minutes, the patient returns to the sitting position. Source: From Fife
TD, Iverson DJ, Lempert T, et al. Practice parameter: Therapies for benign paroxysmal positional
vertigo (an evidence-based review): Report of the Quality Standards Subcommittee of the American
Academy of Neurology. *Neurology* 2008;70(22):2067–2074.

The head is maintained in the same 45-degree left position throughout the
maneuver. The patient is then returned to the sitting position, and the maneuver
is repeated until there is no nystagmus in any position.

Features Shared by the Maneuvers

There are clear similarities in these modified repositioning maneuvers. With
both maneuvers, the patient's head is initially turned 45 degrees to the side,
placing the posterior semicircular canal to be treated in the plane of the subsequent movement. Because the positioning movement with the Epley maneuver is in the sagittal plane, the head is turned toward the affected side, placing
the posterior canal on that side in the sagittal plane, whereas with the Semont
maneuver the head is turned toward the unaffected side, placing the posterior
canal on the affected side in the frontal movement plane. Both maneuvers have
two position changes in the plane of the affected posterior canal moving the

debris sequentially around the canal into the utricle. With both maneuvers, it is a good sign if there is nystagmus in the same direction after each of the two position changes because this indicates that the debris is moving in the right direction toward the utricle. One possible advantage of the modified Semont maneuver is that the entire procedure is performed with the head in the same position without the neck rotation required for the modified Epley maneuver. This may be important in older people with limited neck rotation due to arthritis.

These particle repositioning maneuvers have been shown to be among the most efficacious interventions in all of clinical medicine. Numerous randomized placebo (i.e., sham procedures) controlled treatment trials have been conducted. Trial quality has been rigorously scrutinized independently by the Cochrane Collaboration (Hilton and Pinder, 2004), the American Academy of Neurology Quality Standards Subcommittee (Fife et al., 2008), and a multidisciplinary guideline development panel chosen by the American Academy of Otolaryngology–Head and Neck Surgery Foundation (Bhattacharyya et al., 2008). The results of all the valid randomized controlled trials indicate that the particle repositioning maneuvers have a large effect size in treating patients with BPPV. In these studies, 61–80% of patients treated with a single maneuver had resolution of BPPV compared with only 10–20% of patients in the control groups. Although many more controlled studies have been performed with the Epley maneuver compared to the Semont maneuver, the cure rates seem to be very similar for both maneuvers.

Variations on the Theme

BPPV nearly always results from otoconial debris within the posterior semicircular canal because this is the canal in which it is most easily trapped. If it enters the anterior or horizontal semicircular canals, it typically falls back out and does not become trapped. However, although less common, there are both horizontal and anterior semicircular canal variants of BPPV, and in some cases, the otolithic debris can become attached to the cupula, producing a true cupulolithiasis. As expected, the nystagmus is in the plane of the affected canal; the nystagmus is transient when the debris is freely floating and persistent when it is attached to the cupula. Interestingly, these other canal variants of BPPV can be produced after performing a particle repositioning maneuver for the typical posterior canal variant. As the debris is moved out of the posterior semicircular canal, it can enter the anterior canal from the common crus or it can enter the horizontal canal after it falls into the utricle. The horizontal canal variants of BPPV are important to recognize because the treatment maneuver to get the debris out of the horizontal canal is completely different from those used for the posterior and anterior canal variants.

Horizontal Canal BPPV

Joe McClure was the first to report a horizontal canal variant of BPPV in 1985. He described seven patients who developed positional vertigo and horizontal nystagmus beating toward the ground after turning the head to the side when lying supine (Figure 21.2). The positional nystagmus was strongest when turning toward the affected ear compared to the unaffected ear, consistent with the fact that ampullopetal flow in the horizontal canal results in stronger nystagmus compared to ampullofugal flow (the opposite of the vertical canals). This is how one determines the affected ear, the side with the stronger nystagmus. To explain why the debris did not just fall out of the horizontal canal when the subject lay on the unaffected side (as in Figure 21.2B), McClure speculated that there may be strictures in the membranous canal or the debris is a viscous plug that is sticking to the walls of the canal.

Subsequently, there have been many reports of so-called geotropic (nystagmus beating toward the ground) horizontal canal BPPV. Symptoms are similar to those of the posterior canal variant, but the vertigo attacks last longer and can occur in the upright position, particularly after getting up from supine. The vertigo lasts longer with the horizontal variant because the central feedback (velocity storage) that prolongs the nystagmus response first described by Lorente de Nó (see Figures 12.2 and 12.3) is greater in the horizontal vestibulo-ocular reflex pathways than in the vertical vestibulo-ocular reflex pathways. If a normal subject is accelerated or deaccelerated in the plane of the horizontal canals on a rotating chair (e.g., the ones used by Breuer, Mach, and Crum-Brown), the induced nystagmus lasts approximately three times as long as when the subject's head is tilted to the side so that the rotation occurs in the plane of one of the vertical canal pairs.

As noted previously, the geotropic horizontal canal variant of BPPV often develops immediately after treatment of the posterior canal variant, suggesting that the freely floating debris can enter the horizontal canal immediately after falling out of the posterior canal. It is still somewhat of a mystery why the debris remains in the horizontal canal and does not simply fall out with the normal ear down (see Figure 21.2B). The debris likely does fall out of the canal on its own more easily than when it is in the posterior canal because spontaneous remissions with the horizontal canal variant are much more common than with the posterior canal variant. The average duration of symptoms is much shorter with the geotropic horizontal variant compared to the posterior canal variant.

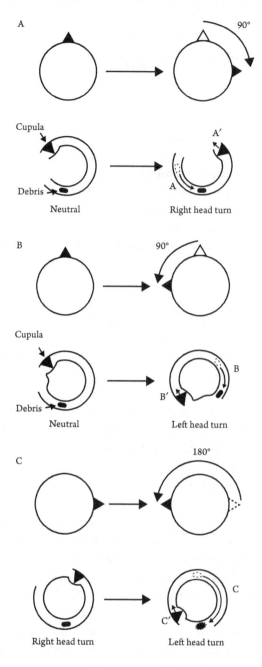

Figure 21.2 SCHEMATIC DRAWING ILLUSTRATING THE MECHANISM OF
GEOTROPIC HORIZONTAL CANAL BPPV INVOLVING THE RIGHT SIDE. (A) The
supine patient turns the head to the right, causing the debris in the right horizontal canal
to move toward the ampulla, which in turn causes excitation of the ampullary nerve firing
and a burst of horizontal nystagmus beating toward the ground. (B) The patient turns the
head to the left, causing the debris to move away from the ampulla, which in turn causes
inhibition of the ampullary nerve firing and nystagmus in the opposite direction again
beating toward the ground. (C) The patient log rolls 180 degrees from the affected right
ear down across to the left ear down to get the debris to roll around the canal into the
utricle. Source: From De la Meilleure G, Dehaene I, Depondt M, et al. Benign paroxysmal positional
vertigo of the horizontal canal. *J Neurol Neurosurg Psychiatry* 1996;60:68–71.

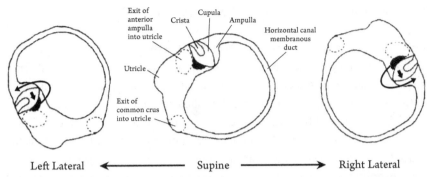

Left Lateral ⟵————————— Supine —————————⟶ Right Lateral

Figure 21.3 SCHEMATIC DRAWING SHOWING HOW A MASS OF DEBRIS ATTACHED
TO THE CUPULA OF THE RIGHT HORIZONTAL SEMICIRCULAR CANAL COULD
PRODUCE APOGEOTROPIC DIRECTION-CHANGING POSITIONAL NYSTAGMUS.
Debris was originally placed on the utricular side of the ampulla. The curved arrows
show where the debris should have been placed on the other side of the cupula. The
small arrows indicate the direction of cupula deviation in right and left lateral positions
regardless of which side the debris is located. Source: From Baloh RW, Yue Q, Jacobson
KM, et al. Persistent direction-changing positional nystagmus: Another variant of benign positional
vertigo? *Neurology* 1995;45:1297–1301.

Numerous repositioning maneuvers have been used to treat the geotropic
horizontal canal variant of BPPV, and eponyms have proliferated but all have the
same basic feature—a roll (log roll or barbeque roll) in the plane of the horizontal canal from the affected ear toward the unaffected ear. The simplest maneuver is to have the supine patient turn the head 90 degrees toward the affected
ear and then rotate across 180 degrees toward the unaffected ear in one motion
(Figure 21.2C). The debris is accelerated toward the utricle and often will be
dislodged with a single rotation. If this is not successful, the patient can sleep on
the side with the unaffected ear down so that gravity will accelerate the debris
toward the utricle. Another simple maneuver to achieve the roll in the horizontal
canal plane is to have the patient sit facing straight ahead and then fall laterally
onto the unaffected ear (similar to the first step of the Brandt–Daroff exercises;
see Figure 20.1) and then turn the head nose down (called the Gufani maneuver
after an Italian otologist). A recent controlled study found that this procedure
was highly effective in curing horizontal geotropic BPPV compared to a sham
procedure (Kim et al., 2012a).

In the early 1990s, my colleagues and I observed several patients who developed another type of horizontal positional nystagmus after undergoing an Eply
maneuver to treat typical posterior canal BPPV—nystagmus beating away from
the ground (apogeotropic) in both lateral positions that persisted for several
minutes before gradually subsiding (Baloh et al., 1995). Although this type of
positional nystagmus was generally considered to be a central sign (originating

from the brain), we believed it must be a variant of BPPV because it occurred immediately after performing an Epley maneuver and it spontaneously resolved over the next several days. In our original report in the journal *Neurology*, we suggested that the nystagmus resulted from cupulolithiasis of the horizontal semicircular canal because recordings of the positional nystagmus were consistent with a constant acceleration (gravity) applied to the cupula of the horizontal canal. We speculated that when the debris re-entered the utricle after the Epley maneuver, it fell up against the cupula of the horizontal canal, where it became lodged against the cupula, similar to Schuknecht's model of cupulolithiasis of the posterior canal (Figure 21.3). The nystagmus gradually decayed over several minutes as the position was held due to central adaptation rather than due to the debris dislodging from the cupula.

Later, it became clear that we had placed the debris on the wrong side of the cupula, just as Schuknecht did in his model of cupulolithiasis of the posterior canal. We came to this conclusion when we converted a patient with apogeotropic persistent positional nystagmus into geotropic paroxysmal positional nystagmus while attempting to dislodge the debris with rapid head turns. The only way this could be explained was that the debris was originally lodged against the horizontal canal cupula on the canal side (rather than the utricular side) and that the exercise dislodged the debris so that it became free floating within the horizontal canal as it typically is with the horizontal geotropic variant (as in Figure 21.2). The patient was then cured of the positional vertigo with a log roll toward the unaffected ear (the side with the lesser geotropic paroxysmal nystagmus). Subsequently, numerous investigators have noted that the persistent apogeotropic horizontal variant of BPPV is converted to the paroxysmal geotropic variant in the process of a successful treatment. What is the best treatment for the apogeotropic variant of BPPV? First, how does one determine the affected side? With the debris attached to the cupula of the horizontal canal, turning the head toward the affected side results in ampullofugal deviation of the cupula, which in turn results in lesser nystagmus than with turning the head toward the unaffected side. In other words, the affected side is the side with lesser apogeotropic nystagmus—the opposite of the geotropic variant. Log rolls toward the unaffected side (the side with the stronger apogeotropic nystagmus) usually work, although it is first necessary to dislodge the debris from the cupula so that it can roll out of the canal. Some recommend vigorous head shaking in the plane of the horizontal canal followed by the log roll or Gufani maneuver. A controlled study found that horizontal head shaking or a reversed Gufani maneuver (fall toward the affected side followed by head turn with nose up) were equally effective for curing the apogeotropic horizontal variant of BPPV compared to a sham maneuver (Kim et al., 2012b).

References

Baloh RW, Yue Q, Jacobson KM, et al. Persistent direction-changing positional nystagmus: Another variant of benign positional nystagmus? *Neurology* 1995;45:1297–1301.

Bhattacharyya N, Baugh RF, Orvidas L, et al. Clinical practice guideline: Benign paroxysmal positional vertigo. *Otolaryngol Head Neck Surg* 2008;139(5 Suppl 4):S47–S81.

Fife TD, Iverson DJ, Lempert T, et al. Practice parameter: Therapies for benign paroxysmal positional vertigo (an evidence-based review): Report of the Quality Standards Subcommittee of the American Academy of Neurology. *Neurology* 2008;70(22):2067–2074.

Hilton M, Pinder D. The Epley (canalith repositioning) maneuvre for benign paroxysmal positional vertigo. *Cochrane Database Sys Rev* 2004;2:CD003162.

Kim JS, Oh SY, Lee SH, et al. Randomized clinical trial for geotropic horizontal canal benign paroxysmal positional vertigo. *Neurology* 2012a;79:700–707.

Kim JS, OH SY, Lee SH. Randomized clinical trial for apogeotropic horizontal canal benign paroxysmal positional vertigo. *Neurology* 2012b;78:159–166.

McClure JA. Horizontal canal BPV. *J Otolaryngol* 1985;14:30–35.

22

Conclusions

Finding a simple cure for the most common cause of vertigo, benign paroxysmal positional vertigo (BPPV), involved many investigators from around the world working more than a century and a half. I chose to focus on five clinical scientists because of the importance of their work and the influence they had on their peers. Their findings have withstood the "test of time" and remain highly relevant. Moreover, these five investigators were interesting people who led very interesting lives. Probably most would agree that the simple cure for BPPV is the "poster child" for success in the field of neurotology. Some would suggest that the credit for discovery of a cure should go to Semont and Epley because they developed and championed the treatment maneuvers. I argue that they simply stood on the shoulders of these five giants who provided the scientific underpinning for developing the maneuvers.

By the end of the 18th century, the detailed anatomy of the inner ear was well described, but it was not until the latter half of the 19th century that it was appreciated that vertigo could originate from damage to the inner ear. Until that time, the inner ear was thought to be exclusively involved with hearing. Based on their appearance, the semicircular canals were thought to be important for localizing sound in space. In the early 19th century, Flourens provided the first real insight into what the semicircular canals might be doing when he systematically cut each of the three canals in pigeons and produced wild gyrations of the animals in the plane of the damaged canal. Although he mistakenly concluded that the semicircular canals somehow controlled head and body movements, his description of the abnormal movements was inspirational to the later work of Ménière and Breuer.

Early knowledge about the balance function of the inner ear came from clinical and experimental observations in animals and humans who had suffered damage to an inner ear. Consider the problems facing the early investigators who were trying to understand how damage to the inner ear causes vertigo and how to treat vertigo. The inner ear is a tiny structure completely surrounded by the hardest bone in the body, the temporal bone (see Figure 1.1). Doctors can easily see the external ear canal and parts of the middle ear through the ear drum on routine examination, but because of its location, the inner ear cannot be seen and is difficult to examine even in postmortem specimens at autopsy. Although simple in concept, clinical assessment of the sense of motion is a difficult task. Sensations originating from the inner ear motion receptors are difficult to differentiate from those originating from tactile and proprioceptive receptors. Because motion sensations originating from the inner ear are more ambiguous than those produced by, for example, auditory or visual stimuli, people have difficulty sensing when the motion begins and ends and the magnitude of the motion. Furthermore, people with damage to the inner ear have difficulty describing the abnormal sensations because these are unlike anything they have previously experienced.

As director of a large deaf-mute institute in Paris, Ménière saw a variety of patients with one-sided hearing loss and vertigo that he likened to the gyrations experienced by Flourens' pigeons. He provided remarkably detailed clinical descriptions of his patients and even complained that some had difficulty providing him the details that he desired. Ménière described patients with features of most of the common inner ear disorders including BPPV, but his main goal was to convince his peers that vertigo could originate from damage to the inner ear and that treatments such as bloodletting were more dangerous than the underlying condition. By contrast, Breuer, though an excellent clinician, did all of his work on animals (mostly pigeons), and there is no evidence that he ever applied his findings to patients with vertigo. Breuer disagreed with Flouren's interpretation of his experiments in pigeons and went on to conclusively show that the inner ear contained sensory receptors that responded to a shear force associated with head acceleration, angular in the case of the semicircular canals and linear in the case of the otolith organs. This shear force resulted in a bending of the tiny hairs projecting into the cupula of the semicircular canals and the otolithic membrane of the otolith organs, which in turn resulted in a change in the firing rate of the sensory nerves supplying these sensory organs. He selectively stimulated each of the inner ear sensory receptors and recorded reflex eye movements, including nystagmus. Breuer's "shear theory" forms the backbone of our current understanding of vestibular physiology.

After the turn of the 20th century, Bárány took the findings in vestibular physiology made by Breuer and colleagues into the clinic and applied them to diagnose patients with vertigo. His caloric test that led to his receipt of the Nobel Prize allowed him to identify one-sided inner-ear damage for the first time. Bárány provided the first clear description of the nystagmus associated with

BPPV, but it was not until the mid-20th century that Hallpike and Dix described the characteristic clinical profile of BPPV. They emphasized that it typically had a benign course and often spontaneously remitted. Hallpike, whose career was accelerated with the early description of the pathology of Ménière's syndrome, later standardized Bárány's caloric test and described the first pathology associated with BPPV. Finally, Schuknecht studied pathological specimens from patients with BPPV at the University of Chicago and also those of Hallpike, and he noted that in some specimens the only remaining semicircular canal was the posterior canal. He would go on to produce an animal model of BPPV in the cat and collect many additional postmortem specimens on his own that supported his cupulolithiasis theory.

Looking back, all the key information for understanding the mechanism of BPPV was known early in the 20th century, but it was not until near the end of the century that a cure was discovered. Wittmaack noted that guinea pigs developed positional nystagmus if their otolithic membranes were dislodged, but Wittmaack's experiments were interrupted by World War I and were never published. Bárány described the characteristic stereotyped appearance of the nystagmus associated with BPPV, and Hallpike provided convincing evidence that BPPV was a benign condition originating from the inner ear, but both misinterpreted the nystagmus as originating from the gravity-sensing utricular macule. Finally, Schuknecht focused attention on the posterior semicircular canal and otolithic debris, but his cupulolithiasis model failed to explain many of the typical features of the nystagmus.

Not surprisingly, early treatment maneuvers based on the cupulolithiasis mechanism were not very effective. Understanding the canalithiasis model was the key to developing effective treatment maneuvers. In retrospect, one the most important publications that should have suggested a simple cure for BPPV was published in a relatively obscure Canadian journal and had few citations (Hall et al., 1979). McClure's model (see Figure 20.2), which used rounded tubes and a water bottle to represent the semicircular canals and utricle and mercury to represent free-floating otolithic debris (the canalithiasis model), clearly showed how debris could enter the canal side of the posterior semicircular canal with the head extended backward and how it could be moved back into the utricle with positioning of the model. However, Hall et al. did not mention the possibility of treatment maneuvers based on McClure's model. There is no evidence that either Semont or Epley were aware of this publication.

Are there lessons to be learned from this historical look at the quest for a cure of BPPV? Certainly one lesson is that clinical science is messy, just like all other areas of science, with missed opportunities, blind allies, serendipitous findings, and academic intrigue. Can we learn from the mistakes of others? Maybe not. But there is some truth in the saying that those who do not know history are destined to repeat it.

Reference

Hall SF, Ruby RRF, McClure JA. The mechanics of benign paroxysmal vertigo. *J Otolaryngol* 1979;8:151–158.

GLOSSARY

Afferent nerve Nerve carrying signals from the periphery to the brain.

Ageotropic Movement directed away from the earth.

Ampulla Dilated ending of the semicircular canal containing the crista and cupula.

Ampullofugal Refers to endolymph movement "away" from the ampulla.

Ampullopetal Refers to endolymph movement "toward" the ampulla.

Bony labyrinth Bony capsule surrounding the membranous labyrinth.

Canalith repositioning maneuvers Treatments intended to move displaced otoconia from the affected semicircular canal to the utricle.

Canalithiasis Mechanism of benign paroxysmal positional vertigo (BPPV) in which otoconia are free floating within the semicircular canal.

Cerebellum Portion of the hindbrain that modulates balance and limb and eye movements.

Cochlea Auditory portion of the labyrinth (inner ear).

Cochlear duct Central duct of the cochlea containing endolymph where the organ of Corti is located.

Crista Sensory epithelium in the ampulla of the semicircular canal containing hair cells that are stimulated by angular acceleration.

Cupula Gelatinous structure filling the ampullae of the semicircular canals.

Cupulolithiasis Mechanism of BPPV in which otoconia are adherent to the cupula.

Dix–Hallpike test Testing procedure in which the patient is moved from a sitting to head-hanging position intended to identify posterior canal BPPV.

Efferent nerve Nerve carrying signals from the brain to the periphery.

Endolymph Fluid inside the membranous labyrinth.

Eustachian tube Tube that connects the middle ear to the back of the throat so that pressure can be equilibrated in the middle ear.

Ewald's laws

> **First** The axis of nystagmus parallels the anatomic axis of the semicircular canal that generated it.

> **Second** Ampullopetal endolymphatic flow produces a stronger response than ampullofugal flow in the horizontal canal.

> **Third** Ampullofugal endolymphatic flow produces a stronger response than ampullopetal flow in the vertical canals.

Geotropic Movement directed toward the earth.

Hair cell Sensory cell that transduces mechanical force into nerve action potentials.

Histological Study of the minute structure of tissues.

Hydrops Distention of the endolymphatic space.

Labyrinth Refers to the inner ear, which includes the cochlea and vestibular organs.

Labyrinthectomy Surgical removal of the labyrinth (inner ear).

Labyrinthitis Infection or inflammation of the labyrinth (inner ear).

Macule Otolith organs containing hair cells that are stimulated by linear acceleration.

Membranous labyrinth The membranous portion of the inner ear that is filled with endolymph.

Myelin Sheaths surrounding nerve fibers providing insulation for rapid electrical transmission.

Nystagmus Reflex eye movements with slow and fast components.

Organ of Corti Sensory epithelium of the cochlea containing hair cells that are stimulated by sound waves.

Oscillopsia Gaze instability with head movement.

Ossicles Middle ear bones (malleus, incus, and stapes) that transmit sound from the tympanic membrane to the oval window of the inner ears.

Osteopenia Decreased calcium in bone.

Otoconia Calcium carbonate crystals embedded within the otolith organs.

Otolith organs Inner ear organs that sense linear acceleration including gravity.

Otoliths Otoconia.

Perilymph Fluid situated between the bony and membranous labyrinth.

Pontine reticular formation Area of the brainstem that generates fast components of nystagmus.

Saccule Labyrinthine cavity containing an otolith organ.

Scarpa's ganglia Contains the nerve cell bodies of the vestibular nerve.

Semicircular canals Circular tubes in the inner ear that sense angular acceleration.

Sensorineural hearing loss Hearing loss due to damage of the cochlea or auditory nerve.

Spiral ganglia   Contains the nerve cell bodies of the auditory nerve.

Stapedectomy   Removal or repair of the stapes, usually in patients with otosclerosis.

Temporal bone   Bone of the skull containing the labyrinth.

Torsion   Rotation of the eye around a roll (center of the pupil) axis.

Tympanic membrane   Ear drum; transmits sound from the external ear to the ossicles of the middle ear, which in turn transmit the sound to the inner ear.

Utricle   Labyrinthine cavity containing an otolith organ.

Vertigo   Dizziness characterized by a sense of movement, usually spinning.

Vestibular   Refers to the vestibular (balance) portion of the labyrinth (inner ear).

Vestibular neurectomy   Surgical section of the vestibular nerve.

Vestibular neuritis   Infection or inflammation of the vestibular nerve.

INDEX

References to figures are denoted with italicized *f*